I Don't Feel Good

I Don't Feel Good

A Guide to Childhood Complaints and Diseases

Jane W. Lammers, EdD, CHES

Suggestions for teachers, parents and other care providers of children to age 10

ETR ASSOCIATES
Santa Cruz, California
1991

ETR Associates (Education, Training and Research) is a nonprofit organization committed to fostering the health, well-being and cultural diversity of individuals, families, schools and communities. The publishing program of ETR Associates provides books and materials that empower young people and adults with the skills to make positive health choices. We invite health professionals to learn more about our high-quality resources and our training and research programs by contacting us at P.O. Box 1830, Santa Cruz, CA 95061-1830.

© 1991 by ETR Associates. All rights reserved. Published by ETR Associates, P.O. Box 1830, Santa Cruz, CA 95061-1830.

10 9 8 7 6 5 4

Printed in the United States of America

Illustrations by Marcia Quackenbush
Design by Ann Smiley and Julia Chiapella

Library of Congress Cataloging-in-Publication Data

Lammers, Jane W.
    "I Don't Feel Good" : a guide to childhood complaints and diseases / Jane W. Lammers.
        p. cm.
    Includes bibliographical references.
    ISBN 1-56071-055-1
    1. Children—Diseases. 2. Child care. 3. Pediatrics—Popular works. I. Title.
    RJ61.L215   1991
    618.92—dc20   91-2630
                                                                CIP

Title No. 584

For John and Ben and all the adults who care about children.

—J.W.L.

Contents

Editor's Preface   ix
Acknowledgments   xi
Introduction   1

Chapter 1.   The Most Common Complaints: The Aches   3
- *I Don't Feel Good*   5
- *Fever*   6
- *Taking a Temperature*   8
- *Stomachache*   10
- *Headache*   15
- *Head Injuries*   17
- *Sore Throat*   17
- *Earache*   20
- *Psychosomatic Complaints*   22

Chapter 2.   Bug Problems: Bites and Stings   25
- *Allergic Systemic Reaction*   27
- *First Aid for Allergic Reactions*   28
- *Mosquitoes, Chiggers and Fleas*   29
- *First Aid for Bites from Mosquitos, Chiggers or Fleas*   30
- *Spiders*   31
- *First Aid for Poisonous Spider Bites*   32
- *Ticks*   32
- *Stings*   33
- *First Aid for Stings*   34
- *Lice*   34
- *Scabies*   37

Chapter 3.   Itchy Problems: Rashes and Sores   41
- *Impetigo*   42
- *Ringworm*   44
- *Conjunctivitis*   46
- *Mouth Lesions*   48

Chapter 4. Catchy Problems: Common Communicable Diseases   51
- *Chickenpox*   53
- *Fifth Disease*   55
- *The Common Cold*   56
- *Influenza*   59

Chapter 5. Preventing Problems: Immunizable Diseases   61
- *Diptheria*   63
- *Tetanus*   65
- *Pertussis*   66
- *Polio*   68
- *Measles*   69
- *Mumps*   72
- *Rubella*   73
- *Haemophilus Influenza Type B (HIB)*   75

Chapter 6. Less Common Problems: Chronic Diseases   77
- *Arthritis*   78
- *Cancer*   80
- *Diabetes*   81
- *Epilepsy*   83
- *Heart Conditions*   84
- *HIV/AIDS*   85

Appendix A. Sample Letters to Parents   89
- *Chickenpox*   90
- *Head Lice*   92
- *Influenza*   94

Appendix B. Over-the-Counter Drugs for Common Skin Conditions   95

Appendix C. Procedure for Keeping an Airway Open   96

Appendix D. Recommended Schedule for Active Immunization of Normal Infants and Children   97

References   99

Suggested Readings   101

Editor's Preface

Having sick children is scary, even for professionals working in the health care system. This book is written to help teachers, parents and caregivers understand and cope with children's illnesses. It's a practical guide to common childhood illnesses.

The author offers technical health and medical information in a way that is easy to understand. She helps adults deal intelligently and sensibly with the reality that all children get sick. Parents can identify with her personal examples as a parent dealing with a sick child. Educators can appreciate the numerous examples she provides that come from her years of teaching teachers and school nurses.

Lists of signs and symptoms help adults identify children's health problems. Suggestions for teachers and caregivers help caring adults identify sick children, control the spread of disease and work with parents to provide appropriate care for sick children. Suggestions for parents offer guidance for treatment of common illnesses, when to contact a physician, what to ask the pharmacist and when to send a recovering child back to daycare or school.

The book will be a valuable reference for adults who care for children. It can help teachers or caregivers decide when to call parents and parents decide when to call the doctor. It includes practical information, such as how to take a child's temperature or what to do about an allergic reaction to an insect bite. Appendixes include sample letters for parents, a list of over-the-counter treatments for skin problems, and first aid to help a child who is having a seizure. The final section of the book provides a list of additional resources and recommended reading.

To ensure that the information provided here was relevant and accurate, the author consulted with pediatricians, school nurses, teachers, daycare providers and other parents. In addition to her numerous personal interviews with these people, two other professionals provided technical reviews of the book.

Dr. Montgomery Kong, a pediatrician in private practice in Walnut Creek, California, and Pat Owen, a staff pharmacist at Longs Drugs in Scotts Valley, California, reviewed and commented on the book from their respective points of view in the health care system. They were concerned with both technical accuracy and the practicality of the information. They helped us address the common questions and concerns that come to them from their patients. This major review process helped the author and editors focus the health information in the book.

Every parent, teacher or caregiver of young children can use the information this book provides. The information can help you work more effectively with health care providers to become partners in the care of children, working together to foster healthy, happy, fulfilled children who will become healthy, happy adults.

Kathleen Middleton MS, CHES
Editor

Acknowledgments

There were many people who made this book a reality and whom I want to thank.

To my husband, John Lammers, thank you for your love, encouragement and professional comments on the book. You've helped make another of my professional dreams come true.

To my son, Ben Lammers, thank you for being my son. You're a great kid and a lot of fun to live with. You've been a great teacher for your mother.

To my mother, Helen Wewer, thank you for being the best mom I could ever have, as well as my biggest fan.

To all my students, teachers and nurses, thank you for sharing your many school experiences and providing me with inspiration for writing the book.

To Judy Boswell, Estelene Duke, Patricia Lewis, Pat Owen and Montgomery Kong, thank you for your thoughtful reviews and comments on the book.

To all my family and friends, thank you for being there with encouragement and support whenever I needed it.

To Netha Thacker, thank you for your patience and support during the writing of the book. Your kind comments helped keep me going during those times when I wondered what I was doing.

And finally, to my friend and editor, Kathleen Middleton, thank you for being you. I admire and respect your creativity, sensitivity and competence. Working with you on this project has been a great experience and a real pleasure.

Introduction

Healthy children are usually happy children. They are a pleasure to be around. They do not often cry or cause sleepless nights. They are eager to learn and to have new experiences. And they are not as expensive or troublesome as sick children. Having healthy children is a dream of every caregiver. Ask any adult who is caring for a sick child! He or she will easily be able to list the advantages of a healthy child.

Although the goal is always to keep kids healthy, all children will get sick. By the time most children are four years old, they are likely to be spending at least part of each day in daycare or early childhood centers. By the time they are five, most children are enrolled in public or private kindergartens. At this time in their young lives, they are interacting with other children in a variety of settings. During this interaction, they are exposed to a variety of bugs and viruses that their bodies may not be able to handle, so they get sick.

For most families, a sick child is at best a major inconvenience and at worst a cause for serious worry. Luckily, by the time children have been around the common early childhood diseases for several years, they do not get sick as often. Their bodies have learned how to fight off infections that once made them ill. In medical terms, this is called *immunity*. For example, many young children have several common colds a year while adults may not have any because they have developed immunity to the many cold viruses that are going around.

Since children are likely to be sick during these early years in school and daycare, teachers, parents and caregivers must learn how to identify when children are sick, what to do for common complaints of illness and how to get sick children well as quickly as possible. Whenever possible, children should be taught to recognize when they are not well and to be very specific about their symptoms, which will help adults identify health problems.

This book discusses the most common childhood conditions that teachers, parents and caregivers see in children between the ages of four and ten. Signs and symptoms of the health problems are described, as well as practical strategies for getting children back to the well state once they are ill. The book also offers guidance in when to seek professional help. In addition, appendixes provide sample letters for parents, a list of over-the-counter medications for common skin conditions, and instructions for emergency treatment for an obstructed airway.

Since the book focuses on the major health complaints of four- to ten-year-old children, caregivers might want to supplement their libraries with additional books on health conditions and health issues of children. A list of suggested resources is provided at the end of the book.

Caregivers may also want to develop basic first-aid skills, so they can be prepared to handle the many first-aid situations that children often experience. The American Red Cross offers an eight-hour course in basic first aid. Contact your local American Red Cross about the many programs.

This book is a collection of common sense ideas both for helping kids stay well and encouraging them to assume personal responsibility for their health. The formative years up to age ten are critical for the development of positive health habits. Everyone who works with children at these ages needs to do everything possible to help create well, happy, fulfilled children who in turn will become well, happy, healthy adults.

Chapter 1

The Most Common Complaints: The Aches

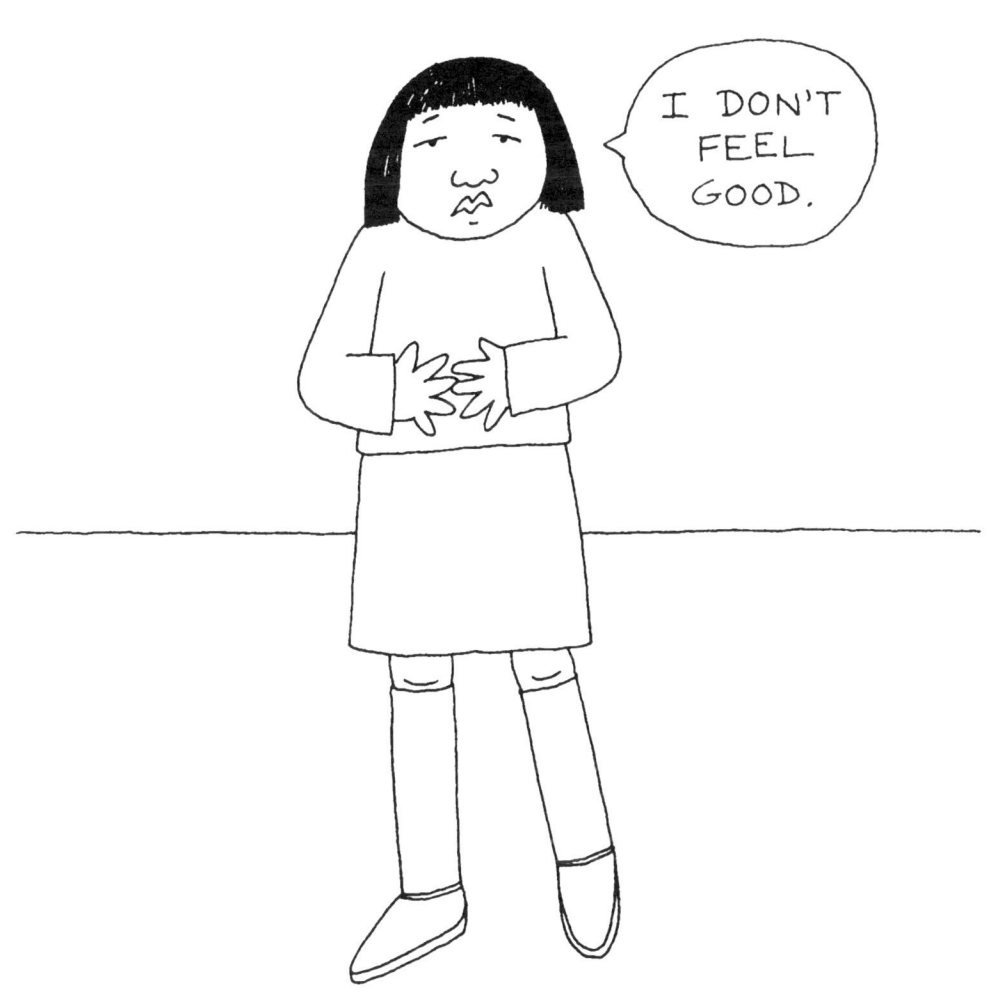

For caring adults who are teachers, parents or caregivers of young children, keeping children healthy is a major concern. To protect children's health, caregivers must be able to listen to and observe children for signs and symptoms that all is not well.

Learning to recognize when a child is getting sick is a skill that can be developed with experience. However, new parents, teachers or caregivers may have to develop the skill quickly. How can we be ready to prevent illness in children? First, we can learn two important clues to children's illnesses. These clues are *signs* and *symptoms. Signs* are things we observe or see; *symptoms* are what children tell us about the way they feel.

Most children are able to tell us they don't feel well by the time they are four years old. When I talk with adults who work with children between the ages of four and ten, I find that the most common health symptoms children report are the *aches:*

- I don't feel good.
- I have a stomachache.
- My head hurts.
- My throat hurts.
- My ears ache.

These symptoms are clues we can use to identify possible illnesses or health problems. When we learn and understand the most basic signs and symptoms of illness, we can prevent many health problems and many of the complications of childhood illness.

Some children do not know how to say they feel bad, so we have to be aware of changes in normal, healthy behavior. Children's behavior can provide clues to their health. A child's activity level may decrease or the attention span shorten. The child may be irritable or sluggish, or the child's eyes may look tired or glassy.

Children who do not verbally communicate their health problems need to be taught to identify their feelings of illness, so they can report future symptoms and speed up the process of getting well.

Parents, teachers and caregivers can learn how to deal with children's minor complaints if they have a general idea of what the complaints might mean. As a teacher or caregiver, you must gather enough information about the complaint to decide if:

- The child will stay at school and you will monitor his or her health the rest of the day.
- You should send a note home reporting the complaint.
- You should call the parents to come get the child.
- You should suggest that the parents take the child to the doctor.

For some conditions, such as fever, daycare or school policies can help you make the decision.

Ultimately, parents are responsible for the health of their children. They must know enough to decide if:

- They can treat the symptom.
- They should call the doctor or take the child to the doctor.
- They should send the child to school.

With just a little basic information, parents can assume responsibility and help children get well much quicker.

I Don't Feel Good

A child who says "I don't feel good" may have a stomachache, a fever, a headache or a number of other problems. My son usually told me he didn't feel good when he was tired. If he had no obvious signs of illness with the "I don't feel good" complaint, I put him down for a short nap. After an hour or two of sleep, he often awoke feeling much better. If you don't know what "I don't feel good" means, encourage the child to be more specific. Ask, "Where on your body do you hurt or not feel good?"

If the response indicates that the complaint is not related to a specific body part, such as the head or stomach, you might suspect fever. Fever causes generalized achiness and an overall "I don't feel good" feeling. If the child complains that a specific body part hurts, see the discussion concerning that ache.

Fever

Many adults think they can tell if a child has a fever by just touching the child's skin. Fever will make the skin feel warmer than usual, but playing outside in the hot sun can also make the skin feel warm. The one sure way to determine if a child has a fever is to use a thermometer to take the child's temperature.

Parents, teachers and caregivers should be skilled at taking a temperature. Many schools provide thermometers, so teachers can take a child's temperature in the classroom before referring the child to the school nurse or parent. Depending on the type of thermometer provided, disposable plastic covers should also be available to cover the thermometer while it's in the child's mouth.

──── *Suggestions for Teachers and Caregivers* ────

✓ If you suspect fever, take the child's temperature. Do not try to guess whether a child has a fever. If the child has a temperature one degree or more higher than normal, arrange for the child to go home or to be separated from the other children. A child who has a fever may be *contagious* (able to spread disease).

Fever is one way the body fights infection. In most cases, a child with a fever should be isolated from other children to avoid spreading disease.

✓ In general, most daycare centers and schools have policies that exclude a child with a fever of 99 degrees or higher. The child may be allowed to return to school when the fever is gone.

Note: Sometimes children with chronic diseases such as arthritis may have fever at a particular time of the day. These children may not have to be excluded from school, but the fever should be reported to parents.

─────────── *Suggestions for Parents* ───────────

✓ If you suspect that your child has a fever, take the child's temperature. Fever temperatures range from low to high, as follows:
low fever—100 to 101 degrees
mildly high fever—102 to 103 degrees
high fever—104 degrees or above

✓ For most low fevers, the fever should be allowed to run its course. Only when the child is prone to febrile convulsions (convulsions occurring during fever, but not due to an infection in the brain) should other measures be taken. Try to keep the child comfortable and encourage her or him to drink lots of fluids. If other symptoms appear with the fever, you may soon understand what is causing the fever.

✓ For mildly high fevers (102 to 103 degrees), try to get the child to drink as much fluid as possible. Some children with fever lose all desire to drink. Offer ice chips if the child won't drink liquids.

✓ Wet a cloth with cool water to wipe the child's body, or place a cool, wet cloth on the back of the neck or on the forehead. You can even splash cool water on the child's head, neck, arms or legs to cool him or her off. Placing the child in a tub of lukewarm water may also lower the temperature. **Do not use alcohol rubs.** Sometimes just taking off most of the child's clothes and putting her or him near a fan will help.

✓ Use acetaminophen to reduce the fever. Common brand names for acetaminophen are Tylenol and Datril. **Do not give aspirin to a child.** Aspirin has been associated with a condition called Reye's syndrome, which affects children. Although rare, this condition can be very serious. Follow the directions on the acetaminophen package for dosage based on age and weight.

Fever

Taking a Temperature

There are various types of thermometers. Some schools provide standard thermometers, while others offer battery-operated, digital-readout thermometers. Taking a temperature with either instrument will provide the same results, but different types of thermometers must be used differently. You must start and finish with a clean thermometer to prevent the spread of infection.

Cleaning the Thermometer

Clean the end of the thermometer that goes in the child's mouth. On a standard thermometer, this is the bulb end. On a digital thermometer, this is the end with the silver tip.

Wipe the end with a tissue that is wet with soap or a sterile cleaning solution, such as alcohol. Repeat the process to be sure the thermometer is clean. Then wipe the thermometer with another tissue that is wet with clean water to remove any soap or disinfectant solution.

Using a Standard Thermometer

- Clean the thermometer.
- Shake down the thermometer to 95 degrees or lower.
- Cover the thermometer with a disposable plastic shield if one is available.
- Place the bulb end of the thermometer under the child's tongue. Tell the child to close his or her lips, but not to bite or chew the thermometer. Wait three minutes.
- After three minutes, remove the thermometer and read the temperature.

Reading the Thermometer

A standard thermometer has a bulb end and a tip end. Hold the thermometer horizontally by the tip end at eye level. The lines on the glass indicate degrees from 94 to 110 degrees Fahrenheit. The short lines between the numbers indicate two-tenths (.2) of a degree. A red line marks normal temperature, which is 98.6 degrees Fahrenheit.

Inside the thermometer is a hollow core containing mercury. The mercury measures the temperature. The point where the mercury falls on the temperature line indicates if the child has a normal temperature or a fever. To read the thermometer, hold the marked side toward you and turn the thermometer until you see where the mercury stops.

- Record the temperature. (Normal is 98.6 degrees Fahrenheit.)
- Clean the thermometer thoroughly, and store in the plastic container provided.

Using a Digital Thermometer

- Clean the thermometer.
- Turn on the thermometer and cover the bulb end with a disposable plastic cover.
- Place the bulb end under the child's tongue until the thermometer beeps or quits flashing.
- Remove the thermometer from the child's mouth and record the temperature.
- Clean the thermometer thoroughly, and store in the plastic container provided.

I Don't Feel Good

Stomachache

✓ For high fevers (104 degrees or higher), use all of the preceding suggestions. Call your physician immediately if the temperature does not drop below 104 degrees. Some children will have convulsions when the fever is high. These convulsions are febrile seizures (fever fits).

✓ If your child has a seizure, make sure that the child will not hit her or his head on anything hard and wait for the seizure to stop. Most seizures will last from a few seconds to a few minutes. If the seizure lasts more than ten minutes, get the child to the doctor. Parents should call the doctor whenever a child has a seizure unless the child has a chronic condition in which seizures occur often and the child is already under medical supervision.

During the seizure, do *not* force anything into the mouth. Keep the child's airway open. (See Appendix C for instructions on proper procedures.) If the child begins to vomit, turn the head to the side, then clear the nose and mouth.

✓ Consult a physician when a child has a temperature higher than 101 degrees for more than two days, even without other symptoms. A physician should also be consulted if a child has a body temperature more than one degree below normal and appears ill. Shock, loss of fluids or excessive sweating may cause lowered body temperature, and any of these can quickly become a serious problem.

✓ Do not send your child back to daycare or school until the fever has been gone for at least 24 hours. A child with fever has a lowered immune system. The child may not be able to fight off infections that other children may have. Children also spread infection when they have fever. Be sure to follow the policies of the school or daycare center regarding fever.

Stomachache

Most stomachaches have emotional rather than physical causes. More than 98 percent of children who are frequently absent from school due to stomachache actually have emotional problems.

Stomachache

Some children get stomachaches when they are not handling stress very well. Stomachaches may be related to school performance or other stressful areas in the child's life. Talking with the child may help you determine if there is some emotional reason for the stomachache.

Of course, you should never assume that a stomachache has emotional causes. Physical causes of stomachaches include minor problems such as overeating, bad food, viruses or flu bugs, constipation, or more serious conditions such as bowel impaction or appendicitis.

When a child complains of a stomachache, ask if the child feels like throwing up or has to go to the bathroom. Vomiting and diarrhea are often associated with stomachaches.

Another question to ask is *where* on the stomach it hurts. (Most kids think their stomachs range anywhere from below the breast to above the pubic bone.) Location may provide another clue to the problem. If the child tells you that the pain begins in the pit of the stomach just below the ribs and increases in severity as it moves to the lower right abdomen, the pain could indicate appendicitis. This type of pain should receive immediate professional attention.

A third question to ask is how the pain feels. Is it sharp like a knife, just general and dull, or nauseating? Sharp, severe pain is usually more serious than general, dull pain. One school nurse described a child in school who was complaining of a severe pain in his stomach. When she asked him when he had last had a bowel movement, he replied that it had been several days. She then suspected a bowel impaction and immediately called the parents to take the child for medical treatment.

Asking these questions will help the child be very specific about the symptoms so that immediate action can be taken to deal with the complaint. Teachers and caregivers should not feel the stomach. If parents choose to feel the stomach, they should touch the area gently. Have the child point to the location of the pain and describe the pain. In general, if a child has a good appetite with a stomachache, the cause is not serious.

I Don't Feel Good

Stomachache

Vomiting:

Vomiting is the way the stomach responds when it is irritated. Sometimes vomiting is a sign of a serious sickness that keeps the stomach from passing food on through the body. Usually, however, it is just a sign that the stomach needs a short rest. To treat vomiting, do not give the child anything to eat or drink for a few hours after the vomiting.

If no vomiting occurs within an hour or two, give the child sips of clear liquids such as Gatorade, flat Seven-up or Sprite, or ice chips if nothing else will stay down. Offer only small amounts. If these liquids are tolerated, add sweetened tea, salty-tasting broth or bouillon, popsicles or jello water. (Mix one teaspoon jello powder to four ounces of hot water, and wait until the mixture is cool enough to drink.)

If no vomiting occurs for eight to twelve hours, add small amounts of foods that are easy on the stomach, such as bananas, applesauce, soda crackers or toast (without the butter). Avoid feeding the child any spicy, fried or greasy food.

If no vomiting occurs for 24 hours, add other foods that the child likes. If vomiting continues for more than 24 hours, call your doctor.

You may send your child back to daycare or school when the child is eating solid foods again.

Diarrhea:

Diarrhea is one way the bowel reacts to sickness. It can be a minor problem that causes little change in normal routine, or it can be a more serious problem that can cause dehydration (loss of body fluids) and death. Diarrhea prevents fluids from being absorbed into the body as they should be. The goal in treatment is to make sure that plenty of fluids are available for the body to function normally.

Diarrhea might be caused by viruses, bacteria, parasites or even stress. Diarrhea is a common side effect of taking some antibiotics. Whatever the cause, treatment is important. Treatment should begin by determining the primary cause of the diarrhea.

If the child is taking antibiotics that cause diarrhea, you may need to call the doctor for advice. Sometimes the medication may be changed, or the doctor may suggest a specific treatment that will control the diarrhea while the child is on medication. For example, unless you are warned not to use milk products with the medication, feeding the child yogurt can help restore the bowel to normal functioning.

If the child has diarrhea because of a virus or some other bug, you will need to encourage the child to drink as much fluid as possible without upsetting the intestinal tract further. Clear liquids may be more easily tolerated.

If the child is losing too much fluid, the skin will not have its normal elasticity. Check the elasticity of the skin by gently gathering a fold of skin on the child's stomach with your fingers. When you let go, the skin should spring back. If it doesn't, the child is probably dehydrated. The child's eyes may also look sunken, and the mouth may be dry. Call your doctor for advice if a child starts becoming dehydrated.

Antibiotics are not prescribed for viral infections since viruses do not respond to such medication. The infection will just have to run its course. However, for bacterial infections or parasites, your doctor may recommend medication to destroy the organisms that are causing the infection.

Continue feeding regular foods to the child. Foods that are usually tolerated well include bananas, rice, applesauce and toast. As with vomiting, avoid giving the child spicy, greasy or fried foods until the diarrhea is over.

Check with your doctor if diarrhea lasts more than four days, if the child is showing signs of dehydration or if there is blood in the stool.

―――― *Suggestions for Teachers and Caregivers* ――――

✓ If the stomachache was caused by a blow to the abdomen and the pain does not go away, call the parents and notify them of the injury.

Stomachache

Suggest that they take the child to a doctor, especially if other more serious symptoms such as increased pain, vomiting, lowered body temperature or shock occur.

✓ If the child with the stomachache does not look sick or does not frown in pain, suggest that he or she lie down or rest with his or her head on the desk for fifteen to twenty minutes.

✓ If the stomachache is not gone within twenty minutes, the child could be sent to the sick room to rest. If necessary, the parents should be called to come get the child. The stomachache is usually not serious if the child does not have any trouble sitting or lying in different positions.

✓ If the stomachache is accompanied by fever, the child should be sent home. A child who is vomiting or has diarrhea probably has a contagious disease and should be sent home.

However, a child may not have to be sent home after only one episode of vomiting. If you suspect that the vomiting was caused by too much exercise after eating or by anxiety, you might observe the child for ten to fifteen minutes. If the child then feels fine, if there is no fever and if no blood was present in the vomit, the child probably does not have to go home.

✓ If a child who has diarrhea is not taking any antibiotics that might cause the condition, the parents should be called to come get the child.

✓ If the stomachache is serious, the pain will get worse with time. Parents should be called to come get the child if this happens.

Suggestions for Parents

✓ If a stomachache is caused by a blow to the abdomen, watch the child for further signs and symptoms of injury. If the pain increases or the child begins vomiting or becomes cold and clammy, contact your doctor immediately.

✓ If the child has a fever with the stomachache, he or she probably has a virus. Treat the symptoms. If you decide to give your child medication, read labels carefully. Some medicines, such as Pepto Bismol, contain aspirin. **Do not give aspirin to children.**

Headache

Another common symptom reported by children is headache. As with the other common complaints, there are numerous reasons for the ache. Most headaches in children are caused by tension or stress. Regular physical exercise and play at school may help reduce the tension and stress that cause the muscles to tense and create a headache. By participating in simple activities that keep the body in good physical condition and that allow the mind to relax, many headaches can be avoided. Other causes of headache include anxiety, fever, allergies, visual problems, head injuries, seizures and even changes in humidity.

When a child complains of a headache, ask where the head hurts and if the child knows why it hurts. If a child tells you that his or her head hurts because he or she was hit on the head, you will need to follow procedures for head injuries. If the child doesn't know why it hurts, you will have to look for other signs and symptoms to determine the cause.

Check the child for other symptoms. Ask yourself the following questions:

- How does the child act? A child who seems to lose energy and wants to go to sleep, vomits or is not conscious may have a serious injury.
- How does the child look? Is the child pale? Are the pupils of the eyes normal? Does the child appear weak?
- How does the child feel? Does the child have a temperature, or is the skin clammy and cold? Is there a bump where an injury might have occurred?
- Does the child complain of a stiff neck or the neck hurting when the chin touches the chest?

Headache

When you have more information, you can make a more informed decision regarding the child's care.

Suggestions for Teachers and Caregivers

✓ If there are no other symptoms, place a warm cloth on the back of the neck and have the child rest, head down on the desk, for fifteen to twenty minutes. If the child doesn't feel better, send him or her to the sick room to lie down. If the headache progresses or other symptoms occur, call the parents to come get the child.

✓ Send children with headaches accompanied by fever or vomiting to the sick room, and call their parents to come get them. Many children complain of headache when they have a viral or bacterial infection.

✓ If the child is reporting frequent headaches while at school, you may want to have a conference with the parents to discuss the problem.

✓ Do not give any medication at school or the daycare center for a headache. Only the parent should give medication to the child.

Suggestions for Parents

✓ Determine a possible cause for the headache if you can. Most headaches are caused by tension and stress (yes, young children can have tension headaches). If you suspect that the headache is due to stress, talking with your child might help you understand some of his or her anxieties and fears. (See the discussion of psychosomatic complaints under stomachaches.)

✓ If the headache is caused by an earache, toothache, sore throat, common cold or a more serious infection, those complaints should be treated to relieve the headache. If fever is present, the child probably has some kind of infection.

> **Head Injuries**
>
> • Observe the child. If there is a bump on the head, use an ice pack to reduce the swelling.
>
> • If the child has lost consciousness when injured, cannot remember the accident, has a seizure, becomes irritable or sluggish, vomits, has irregular breathing or heartbeat, has irregular pupils or complains of severe head pain, the child should be seen by a doctor as soon as possible.
>
> • If none of these symptoms occur, watch the child for the rest of the day. If a child at school has had a minor headache from a bump on the head, notify the parents at the end of the day, so they can continue to watch the child for 24 hours.

✓ When no other symptoms are present, treat headaches with rest and a warm cloth on the back of the neck. If you use a pain reliever, remember to choose acetaminophen and **not aspirin**.

✓ The child may return to school when the headache is not associated with fever, vomiting, head injuries or an infectious disease. Children should be taken to the doctor for frequent headaches that have no known cause.

Sore Throat

Sore throat is another common complaint of children. Sore throats are often combined with fever, headache or earache. Children get two types of infectious sore throats—viral and bacterial. If the sore throat is viral, medication does not affect the illness but may prevent secondary infection. A secondary infection occurs when the body's immune system cannot fight

I Don't Feel Good

Sore Throat

off other diseases because it is busy fighting off the viral infection. Bacterial sore throats are often caused by a germ called *streptococcus*. This condition is usually called *strep throat*.

Some parents believe that tonsils are responsible for sore throats. Today, we know that is not true. Tonsils are lymphoid tissue and are designed to help the body fight off infection. The tonsils are largest in children between the ages of four and seven because their bodies are fighting off many colds and upper respiratory infections.

Only when the tonsils are so large that they interfere with the child's breathing, eating or swallowing, or the child has recurring abscesses of the tonsils should they be removed. All of these conditions are rare, and parents should seriously discuss the issue with their child's physician if a tonsillectomy is recommended.

Sore throats may also be caused by breathing with the mouth open. Some children who have allergies or sinus problems cannot breathe normally through their noses, because the nasal passages are swollen. These children become mouth breathers. If the humidity is low, the irritation to the throat is greater.

Sore throats are more common in the winter when many families use woodburning stoves and heating systems that take humidity from the air, but do not provide for additional humidity in the home. Sore throats caused by mouth breathing or sleeping with an open mouth are usually only reported in the morning and are gone after a few hours.

If a child complains of a sore throat, ask the child how she or he feels. Look for other signs and symptoms of illness. Find out when the sore throat started. Was it sudden? Is the throat sore only in the morning, or has it been hurting for several days? Gather as much information as you can.

Suggestions for Teachers and Caregivers

✓ If there are no other symptoms and the sore throat is causing only minor pain, not much can be done. Gargling with salt water (one teaspoon in one cup of warm water) may relieve the pain temporarily. Watch the child for the rest of the day to see if anything else develops.

✓ If symptoms such as fever, difficulty in swallowing, drooling or difficulty in breathing occur with the sore throat, notify the parents. Suggest that they take the child to a physician. A throat culture (swabbing) may be done to determine if the sore throat is viral or bacterial.

✓ The child may return to school if he or she does not have fever and the serious symptoms are gone.

Suggestions for Parents

✓ If the pain of the sore throat is minor and there are no other symptoms, have the child gargle with salt water (one teaspoon in one cup of warm water). Watch for any other symptoms.

✓ If the sore throat occurs only in the morning during the winter, check the humidity in the home. Using a cool-mist humidifier in the room where the child is sleeping can help prevent a dry, irritated sore throat in the morning.

✓ Painful sore throats that come on suddenly and are accompanied by other symptoms such as fever, drooling, or difficulty in breathing or swallowing should be examined by a physician. The doctor may choose to take a throat culture to determine the cause of the sore throat.

✓ If the infection is viral, no medication may be prescribed. All that can be done is to treat the symptoms. Children's doctors might suggest acetaminophen, a pain reliever, or cold medications to control any drainage from a cold or allergy that may irritate the throat. Gargling with salt water and using a humidifier may also help. (Be sure to clean the humidifier frequently as recommended by the manufacturer to avoid spreading mold that grows when water sits in a container for any length of time.)

✓ If the infection is bacterial, antibiotics will probably be prescribed.

Follow all the directions in taking the medication, *even if the symptoms are gone before the medicine is finished.* A more serious infection may occur if medication is stopped too early.

✓ An untreated strep throat may lead to serious complications such as a throat abscess or rheumatic fever. Rheumatic fever causes painful swollen joints and unusual skin rashes. The heart valves may also be damaged.

✓ Complications from strep throat can be prevented by taking antibiotics as prescribed by a doctor. In other words, with questionable sore throats, going to the doctor is your best course of action.

✓ You may send your child back to school when the fever and more serious symptoms are gone.

Earache

Almost all children will experience an earache at some time. Earaches can be caused by ear infections, putting things in the ear, cutting new teeth, injuries or from dirty water that gets in the ear when swimming. Ear infections, which cause most of the complaints, are usually a complication of a cold or respiratory infection.

When the tube that connects the middle ear with the nasal passages (nose) is swollen or closed, fluid and pressure build up in the child's middle ear, resulting in an ear infection. For some children, ear infections are a chronic problem throughout their childhood years.

For chronic ear infections, ear tubes (ventilation tubes) may be inserted in the ear drum to provide adequate air circulation in the middle ear. The air flow helps the ear to heal and prevents the middle ear from being closed. Ear infections do not usually occur unless the middle ear is closed. Although some children have many ear infections as small children, such infections often decrease once they start school.

Sometimes children will put pencils, peas, small gravel or sharp objects in their ears. When you ask them what they are doing, many children say they are trying to scratch an itchy ear or just playing around to see what happens. An elementary principal I know reported that kindergartners were putting small pebbles in their noses to see if they could blow them out. A few parents had to be called to take their children to the doctor to fish out the stuffed pebbles. Younger children should be taught not to put objects in their ears or noses, or they may try unusual things to see what happens and end up with big problems.

If a child complains of an earache, ask the following questions:

- When did the ear start hurting? Did it suddenly start hurting, or was it hurting earlier?
- Has the child been swimming recently?
- Does the child know why his or her ear hurts? If the child put a pencil in his or her ear or was hit on the head, the ear may be damaged.
- How does the ear ache? Is it constant pain, sharp pain or dull pain? Does the ear itch?
- Are there any other symptoms? Does the child's throat hurt? Is his or her nose stopped up? If the earache occurs with other symptoms, the child may have an infectious disease or allergies.

Look for signs of an ear problem. Check to see if there is a discharge coming out of the ear or if the ear is red and irritated.

Suggestions for Teachers and Caregivers

✓ If there are no other signs or symptoms with a minor earache, watch the child the rest of the day. Teachers or caregivers should send a note home or call the parents to let them know about the complaint.

✓ Contact the parents to come get the child if the earache causes any of the following signs or symptoms: severe or sharp pain, fever, a bloody discharge from the ear, or a white or yellow smelly discharge from the ear. Suggest that the child be seen by a doctor.

Psychosomatic Complaints

―――――――― *Suggestions for Parents* ――――――――

✓ Take your child to the doctor if he or she has any of the following signs or symptoms of an ear problem:
   bloody discharge from the ear
   fever
   ear pain that is sharp and constant
   a white or yellow smelly discharge from the ear

✓ The doctor will be able to look in the ear with a special instrument to see if the ear drum is bulging or has burst. If the ear is infected, the child may need to take antibiotics and/or ear drops to help heal the ear. Do not send your child back to school until the symptoms are gone.

✓ For minor earaches, watch the child for other symptoms. If the ear is itchy, the child may have swimmer's ear or some kind of skin infection in the ear. Ask your doctor for suggestions for treatment, or consult a book such as *Taking Care of Your Child,* by R. H. Pantell, for home remedies.

✓ If no other symptoms occur, you may want to give acetaminophen for pain relief. Be sure to follow directions on the bottle or package. Remember—**no aspirin should be given to children.**

Psychosomatic Complaints

Sometimes children say they are sick, but they really aren't. A child may say, "I don't feel good, my stomach hurts," or, "My head hurts," but there may not be any physical cause for the ache. Medical authorities label this illness a *psychosomatic complaint*—a condition of the body that is caused by the mind. The pain is very real, but the cause is emotional.

There are many reasons for children to report illness when they aren't really sick. Some possible reasons include:

❧ The child might be having a hard day and need a break.

- The child might not want to deal with a problem in the home or school and won't have to if he or she is sick.
- The child may need extra attention, and the only way to get it is to get sick.
- The child might be having to do something he or she does not feel able to do, and the only way to get out of it is to get sick.
- The child may have been taught that people who are sick are not expected to take care of responsibilities such as going to school or doing homework.

Whatever the cause, these complaints are very real to children, and adults must decide how to handle the complaint.

If you've ruled out physical causes for the complaint, you may need to help the child deal with stress. Children can learn to use exercise or relaxation activities to help them cope with stress. *Smiling at Yourself: Educating Young Children About Stress and Self-Esteem,* by Allen Mendler (Network Publications, 1990), suggests activities to help children relieve stress. The book is also useful for helping children develop self-esteem.

As caring adults, you play a large role in maintaining children's health and well-being. You have to be able to determine when and if they are sick and what to do about it if they are. To help you make the best possible decisions, one of your major responsibilities is to teach children how to communicate to you when they might be sick.

If we help children understand cause and effect, we help them associate a pain or an ache (a specific symptom) with a possible reason for the problem. In the future, children will be more likely to provide us with more information about their conditions. Then we can help them feel better more quickly.

We also teach children to become responsible for their health. As they develop and mature, they will be better able to take care of themselves and, in turn, their future children.

Chapter 2

Bug Problems: Bites and Stings

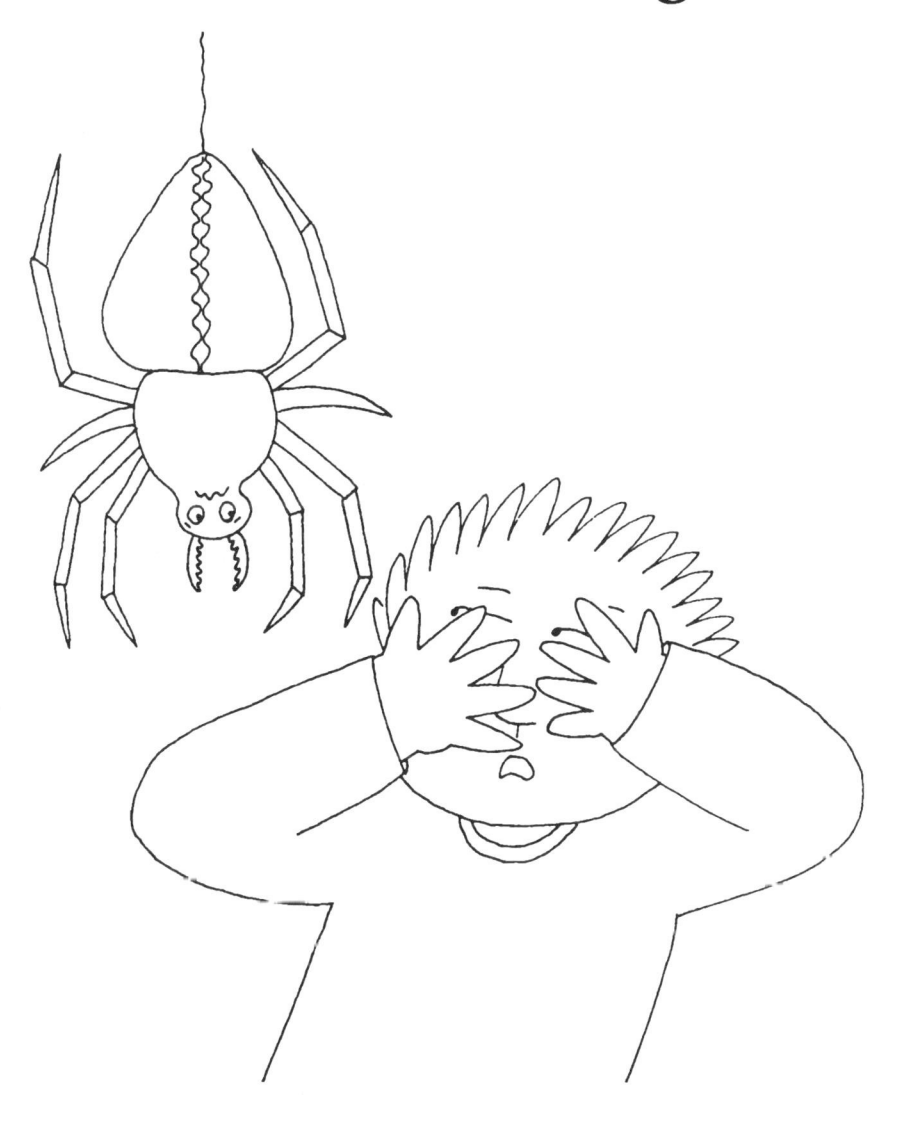

The wonderful world of nature is fun for children to explore. Many of us encourage our children to spend time outside, where they are very likely to come into contact with some of those wonderful bugs and small critters that bite and sting and cause pain and itching. Children also play with other children, so they can easily share bugs like lice and scabies. However, knowing that skin problems are common is of little comfort when your child has a problem.

One teacher who was taking a college class from me described her family experience with head lice. When she picked up her child one evening from daycare, she was told that she would need to check him for head lice. Several children in the daycare center had already been sent home with head lice. She went home and carefully separated each hair on her son's head to be sure there weren't any of those nits that would indicate he had been infested. She repeated this procedure every night until one night she saw some nits.

She reminded herself of what we had discussed in class about dealing with lice and other pest diseases. "Don't panic. Just deal with the problem if it arises." She purchased an over-the-counter medication, followed the directions for treatment, washed all of her son's bedding and towels and put all his stuffed animals in plastic bags for two weeks. She reported that the crisis was soon over, but not without some difficult moments.

Some of the problems we have to face as parents, teachers or caregivers can make us feel squeamish, but we all know that someone has to take care of the child. The more we learn about the conditions, the less afraid we are to deal with them.

So my first word of encouragement is, if your child has some kind of skin problem, don't panic! Review the signs and symptoms of the most common problems and try to figure out what might be wrong. Then follow recommended treatment for taking care of the problem. If all else fails, call or visit your doctor for help.

Many skin problems of children are caused by bites and stings from small insects and other critters. Examples of the more common bugs include mosquitoes, chiggers, fleas, spiders, ticks, bees or wasp-like insects, lice and scabies. Some of these are more prevalent in certain parts of the United States, and some may cause a major problem in your location.

Bug problems can be quite unnerving for any caregiver to handle. In some cases, the bug is present and getting rid of the bug solves the problem. Remember, your reaction to the sight of bugs will be scrutinized by young children. I have a friend who couldn't understand why her son was so traumatized by the sight of spiders. My friend then saw her son's caregiver react hysterically at the sight of a spider. This reaction certainly had been communicated to her young charge.

Actual bug bites may involve very serious physical reactions to the injected venom. Knowing how to apply basic first-aid treatment may be very important in preventing serious complications to the overall health and well-being of our children.

With bites or stings, the primary concern of parents, teachers and other caregivers is the child's reaction to the skin irritation. For most children, the first response is pain or itching or both. Then the body usually responds with a small bump at the place on the skin where the child was bitten or stung.

Allergic Systemic Reaction

More serious reactions range from multiple hives around the bite or sting to serious swelling in the throat that causes difficulty in breathing. Such a serious response is called an *allergic systemic reaction*. If the reaction is not treated quickly, the child may lose consciousness and even die.

When I was very young, I was stung by a wasp. As with most children, my first response was to cry because of the pain of the sting. When I showed my mother what had happened, she saw that hives had developed all over my body. I was having a more serious reaction to the sting than most people.

I Don't Feel Good

Allergic Systemic Reaction

> ### First Aid for Allergic Reactions
>
> • Apply a paste of baking soda or meat tenderizer and cover the bite with an ice pack as soon as possible. Look for signs and symptoms of a serious reaction.
>
> • If you are not prepared to treat a serious reaction, take the child to the nearest emergency room or medical facility. ***Do not delay getting treatment for the child.***
>
> • Parents of children with known allergic reactions should notify daycare or school officials of the child's sensitivity. Parents should also provide emergency kits containing injectable epinephrine and training in administering the treatment in emergencies. Some physicians recommend that children with extreme hypersensitivity wear medic alert bracelets or tags for their protection in case of an emergency.

Since that first sting, I have been stung two more times. With each sting, I had a more serious response. I now keep medication with me in my first-aid kit to prevent a reaction that could be fatal if I am ever stung again. Fortunately, few people have a serious allergic reaction the first time they are stung, although it is not uncommon for a serious reaction to occur after being stung multiple times, such as by a swarm of yellow jackets.

How do you know if a child is having an allergic reaction? You might suspect there is a problem if the child displays any of the following signs and symptoms.

Signs and Symptoms:
- flushed skin
- difficulty in breathing
- wheezing, as in asthma

- fainting
- hives or skin rash
- generalized swelling, especially under the tongue or in the mouth
- sneezing or coughing
- puffy face, mouth or eyelids

Since most bites or stings do not cause serious reactions, minor first aid will usually be all that is necessary to take care of the problem.

Mosquitoes, Chiggers and Fleas

When mosquitoes, chiggers and fleas bite, these small insects release a chemical under the skin that usually causes itching. First-aid treatment is designed to control the itching from the bite and to prevent a secondary infection. If the child scratches the bite, he or she is likely to break the skin and create an open sore that may be susceptible to other infections.

In most of the world, mosquitoes are known to transmit many diseases to humans and animals. In the United States, however, proper sewage control and draining of swampy areas have greatly lessened the danger from diseases spread by mosquitoes. Many communities also spray insecticides frequently during the summer months to control the spread of mosquitoes. Although Americans do not usually suffer from the many fevers that are spread by mosquitoes, we still have problems with mosquito bites and the consequent itching.

Chiggers or redbugs are small red mites that bite. The bites usually occur around the waistline and ankles and cause a lot of itching. The best protection from these small pests is to use insect repellent and wear clothing over the most susceptible parts of the body. Washing as soon as possible after exposure can cut down on some of the bites. Bathing in a bathtub of water mixed with one capful of chlorine bleach or swimming in a chlorinated pool can also help. Some people reduce chigger bites by applying rubbing alcohol to the skin after being exposed to grass and trees that may have chiggers.

First Aid for Bites from Mosquitoes, Chiggers or Fleas

• Wash the bites with soap and water. Dry the area and put a baking soda bandage on the bite for thirty minutes to one hour. To make a baking soda bandage, wet the center of a Band-Aid with a few drops of water and spread on a little baking soda. If you don't have a Band-Aid, mix a small pinch of baking soda with water and make a small pack on the bite.

• If there are multiple bites, give the child a bath in 1/2 cup of baking soda or oatmeal per tub of warm water. The soda or oatmeal bath will help control the itching. Initially the heat of the bath may temporarily increase the itching, but that's good.

The chemical that the bug injected into the skin caused the body to respond to the bite by producing a substance called *histamine*. Histamine causes swelling. When released, it causes itching. Heat releases histamine, and itching will increase temporarily. But after the bath, because histamine has been released from the cells, little of it will be present to cause itching. The child should have relief from the itching for several hours at a time. The hotter the bath or shower, the more histamine will be released, and the longer the relief from itching.

• Calamine lotion or topical over-the-counter medications with cortisone sometimes help relieve itching. For severe itching, some over-the-counter antihistamines may also be useful. Antihistamines tend to make the child sleepy, so they are most useful at nighttime.

Fleas can also cause bites that itch intensely. With so many animals living both inside and outside today's homes, having fleas in the house seems normal. Fleas are tiny insects that feed on warm-blooded animals. They are not particular about which type of warm-blooded animal they feed on, so humans may suffer from flea bites. The amount of itching caused by the bites varies for each person.

Spiders

Spiders are another type of bug that can cause skin irritations, but serious problems are rare. In the United States, the spiders that cause the most serious problems are the black widow and the brown recluse. Of the two spiders' bites, the black widow's is the most serious.

The **black widow** is a black spider with a characteristic red or yellow hourglass-shaped mark on the underside of the abdomen. It is usually found in dark corners of barns, garages and basements and in piles of stone and wood. The black widow bite is often painless. Shortly after the bite, however, the following signs and symptoms may occur.

Signs and Symptoms:

- two tiny red spots at the site of the bite
- severe abdominal pain and generalized large muscular rigidity
- difficulty in breathing
- nausea, vomiting, headaches, perspiration and extreme restlessness

The **brown recluse** spider is slightly smaller than the black widow spider. It has a dark brown violin-shaped mark on the upper back and head. Its bite may cause pain, or the bites may be painless at first and not even be noticed. Brown recluse bites, if not treated, can cause the bitten area to slough off, leaving an open hole in the skin down to the bone. As the name suggests, this spider prefers dark places where it is seldom disturbed—such as old trash piles, attics, storerooms and closets. It will only bite when annoyed or surprised. The following signs and symptoms may indicate a brown recluse spider bite.

Signs and Symptoms:

- pain within two to eight hours after the bite
- blister, swelling and redness at the site of the bite
- rash, nausea, chills, fever, cramps or joint pain

- blister develops into an indented ulcer
- tissue around bite dies and sloughs off

Bites from poisonous spiders are serious for children. If you suspect that a child has been bitten by a poisonous spider, it is helpful, if the spider is still around, to kill it or put it in a jar. You should take the spider to the doctor or emergency room so that it can be properly identified. Then follow recommended first-aid procedures immediately.

First Aid for Poisonous Spider Bites

- Wash bite with alcohol or hydrogen peroxide.
- Apply ice or cold packs to the bite.
- Keep the child quiet.
- If the child is at daycare or school, call the parents immediately and notify them of the bite. Parents should take the child to the doctor or nearest emergency medical facility as soon as possible, especially if there is a severe reaction to the bite.

Ticks

Ticks are another pest that can cause skin problems as well as carry diseases to humans. They are bloodsucking bugs that attach themselves to warm-blooded animals to feed. Both animals and humans suffer from tick bites.

Proper reactions to tick bites include taking the tick off of the body and treating the bite. Ticks should be removed as soon as possible after the bite. Carefully, without crushing the tick, place a tweezers close to the skin and using gentle steady pressure, remove the tick. Protect your hands with gloves, cloth or a tissue when removing the tick. If the head is left under the skin, soak the area of the tick bite with warm water twice a day. Monitor the child for signs and symptoms of diseases that are spread by ticks.

Two major tick-borne diseases are Lyme disease and Rocky Mountain spotted fever. If a child develops any of the following signs or symptoms after being bitten by a tick, parents should take the child to the doctor for diagnosis and treatment.

Signs and Symptoms:

- flu-like symptoms (fever, chills, and headache)
- rash or a ring-shaped red spot like a bull's eye that grows larger every day (Lyme disease) or a rash on the extremities (hands and feet, including the palms and soles) that spreads to all parts of the body (Rocky Mountain spotted fever)
- stiff neck and difficulty concentrating
- pain and swelling in the joints

If a child develops signs of serious infection from a tick bite, appropriate antibiotics may be necessary to prevent permanent damage and even death from the disease.

Stings

Stings by flying insects such as honeybees, wasps, hornets or yellow jackets can also create skin problems for children. Stings from these flying insects usually cause pain where the sting occurred on the body. Such stings can be very dangerous, and parents, teachers and other caregivers should watch for any of the signs of a serious reaction to the sting. (See the description of an allergic reaction at the beginning of this chapter.)

With the exception of the honeybee, flying insects can sting a person repeatedly, injecting small amounts of venom into the body each time a sting occurs. The honeybee will only be able to sting once before it loses its barbed stinger. Since venom can continue to be injected into the body

---

First Aid for Stings

• Unless the child is having an allergic reaction, remove the stinger, if present, by gently scraping it out with a sharp object such as a knife blade, a fingernail or a stiff piece of paper. Credit cards also work well. ***Do not*** grasp the stinger with fingernails or a tweezer, because this forces the remaining venom into the skin.

• Make a baking soda bandage (or use meat tenderizer instead of baking soda). Place it on the sting for thirty minutes to one hour. The baking soda, an alkaline substance, will neutralize the acid in the venom. Meat tenderizer is an enzyme that will break down the protein in the venom and help dissolve the bump from the sting.

• Watch for signs of an allergic reaction. Allergic responses are more likely to occur if the child was stung more than once or had a serious reaction to a prior sting.

---

if the stinger is left behind, you should properly remove the stinger as quickly as possible after a child has been stung.

Any time a child is stung at daycare or school, the parents of the child should be notified. If there is an *allergic reaction,* contact the parents immediately. (Follow suggestions provided at the beginning of this chapter.) For cases not involving an allergic reaction, notify the parents after you have administered first-aid treatment.

Lice

Two other bugs that commonly create skin problems for children are lice and scabies. A child infected with these bugs should be isolated from other children until treatment occurs.

Head lice create a lot of anxiety. People with head lice feel very uncomfortable because they have these bugs crawling around in their hair, and people around them tend to associate the problem with uncleanliness. When lice were common among people who did not bathe regularly because of lack of indoor plumbing, head lice were thought to affect only those who did not practice good hygiene. Today, we know that anyone can get head lice, regardless of how clean she or he is. Especially during the winter months, many schools and daycare centers report cases of head lice.

Lice are bloodsucking insects that feed on humans. There are three types of lice that can infect people—head, body, and pubic lice or crabs. Head and pubic lice spend their life cycle on the skin of the human host. Body lice live in the clothing and only come to the skin to feed. The insects are tiny, although they can be seen with the naked eye if one has good eyesight. Most people can see them with a magnifying glass.

Head lice are the most prevalent lice in children. Most daycare centers and elementary schools will have at least one case of head lice a year, if not more. Head lice are transmitted by direct contact with an infected person or by indirect contact with the infected person's belongings, such as combs, brushes, scarves, coats or headgear.

To prevent the spread of lice, children should be taught how to maintain personal cleanliness. They should also be taught not to share personal items such as combs, brushes, hats and scarves. Clothing should not be hung in closely crowded racks, unfortunately a common practice in many schools.

Each individual female louse lays about three or four nits (eggs) a day during her thirty-day life cycle, for a total of about one hundred nits. The nits are firmly attached to the hair shafts of the host animal (the child). The nits will usually hatch in seven to ten days. Within two weeks, the immature lice become mature, capable of beginning a new cycle.

The most common sign of head lice is the presence of nits. The nits will look like tiny white bumps on the hair strands. You might suspect dandruff, except dandruff can be easily removed from the hair shaft while lice nits cannot be.

Lice

Signs and Symptoms:

- presence of lice (you may need a magnifying glass to see the lice)
- itching
- small red bites resembling a rash on the scalp and behind the ears and neck

―――― *Suggestions for Teachers and Caregivers* ――――

✓ If a child has head lice, separate the child from the other children without embarrassing the child.

✓ Contact the parents to take the child home for treatment.

✓ Check all the other children in the classroom for head lice.

✓ Exclude the child from school until the hair has been properly treated and all the nits are removed. (Some schools require children to bring the box that contained the lice treatment with them to show school officials upon the children's re-entry to school.)

✓ Recheck the child's hair in seven to ten days to determine if the child has been reinfected.

―――――― *Suggestions for Parents* ――――――

✓ If your child has head lice, remain calm and treat the condition.

✓ Purchase an over-the-counter medication for lice. Lice medications come in the form of shampoos or creme rinses. (See Appendix B for examples.) Follow the directions as recommended on the label.

✓ Comb out all the nits with the fine-tooth comb that is provided in most lice treatment packages. If one is not provided, you will need to purchase a fine-tooth comb to comb out the nits. The major reason lice recur is because all the nits are not combed out.

✓ At the same time you treat the hair, wash all bed linens, towels, brushes and head apparel in hot, soapy water.

✓ Place all objects that cannot be washed, such as stuffed animals, in plastic bags for ten days.

✓ Check other members of your household for head lice and treat them if necessary.

✓ Recheck your child's head for the presence of lice or nits for the next ten days. Some treatments may need to be repeated a second time.

✓ In severe cases of lice, consult your physician. There are stronger prescription medications that you may need to use.

✓ You may send your child back to school after the hair has been treated and when all the nits are gone.

Scabies

Scabies, another itchy pest condition, is caused by a mite similar to the chigger. As with lice, in the past people were incorrectly thought to have the condition because they were unclean. Anyone can get scabies, and many daycare centers and schools report epidemics during the winter months. Caregivers should avoid embarrassing a child who contracts scabies and think about treating the condition.

Scabies is contracted by direct contact with a person who has scabies or by indirect contact with infected clothing or bedding. Initial symptoms do not appear until about two to six weeks after infection with the scabies mite. The following are the most common signs and symptoms of scabies.

Signs and Symptoms:
- intense itching, usually more severe at night
- raised grayish lines, called burrows, in the creases of the body, i.e.,

Scabies

- between the fingers, around the stomach, in the armpit, behind the knees
- redness, swelling and blisters developing after scratching the burrows
- presence of the mite (If you can locate a burrow, you may be able to see the mites with a magnifying glass.)

Suggestions for Teachers and Caregivers

✓ If a child has the symptoms of scabies, call the parents to take the child home for treatment.

✓ Exclude the child from daycare or school until the day after treatment.

✓ Observe other children in the class for signs and symptoms of scabies. Notify parents if you suspect other children are infected.

Suggestions for Parents

✓ If you suspect that your child has scabies, take him or her to a physician. If a diagnosis of scabies is made, the physician will prescribe a medication that will kill the mite. Follow all the directions for treatment.

✓ Use calamine lotion for the itching, or soak the child in a tub with baking soda. In severe cases of itching, an over-the-counter antihistamine may be helpful. Follow the directions for dosages according to the age and weight of the child.

✓ If the condition is not gone within a week, a second treatment may be necessary.

✓ If you have difficulty getting rid of the scabies, call your physician for advice.

✓ You may send your child back to school the day after treatment, or as determined by policy developed by individual schools or daycare centers.

All parents, teachers and caregivers are likely to encounter children who will experience bites and stings. Knowing the basic signs and symptoms and ways of dealing with the problem can alleviate a lot of the anxiety for both the child and the caregiver.

Chapter 3

Itchy Problems: Rashes and Sores

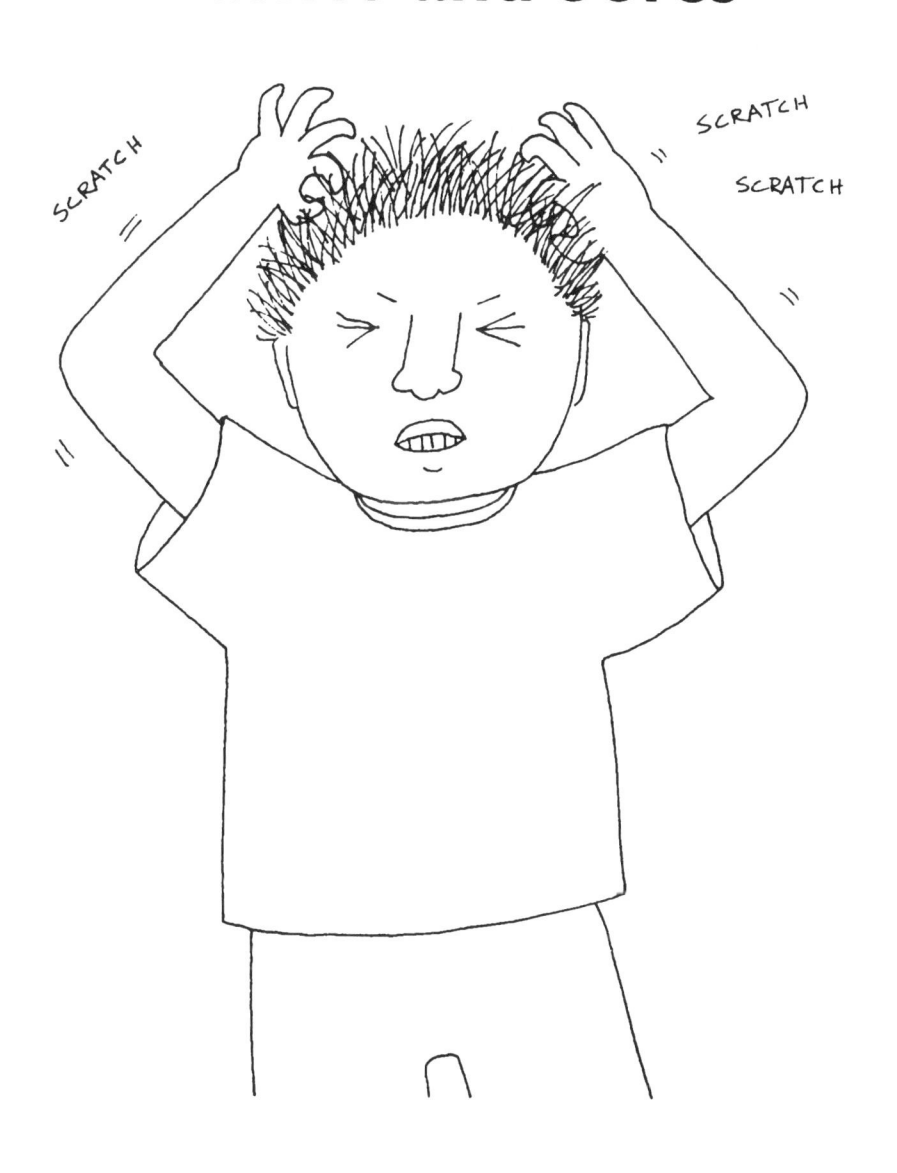

Some skin problems children have are not caused by insects or bugs. Viral or bacterial skin infections may cause skin rashes and lesions. These skin conditions may occur if a bite or sting becomes infected, or they may be caused by the many organisms that can infect the body when the immune system is weak.

Many of these skin infections are contagious, and preventing the spread of the infection is an important part of treatment. Teach children to wash their hands frequently. Good hygiene can often help more to control the disease than antibiotics.

The most common skin conditions seen in children in daycare centers and schools are impetigo, ringworm, conjunctivitis (or pink-eye) and mouth lesions.

Impetigo

Impetigo is an extremely contagious skin disease, most often seen in infants and children. The infection is often caused by a streptococcal bacterium that causes sores or lesions on the skin. Many times the sores begin with cold sores or insect bites that become infected.

Impetigo is spread by direct contact with the sores. When a child has impetigo, scratching can spread the sores to other parts of the body. The sores can spread until they become dry. Impetigo is more common during the summer months. It occurs more often in warm, humid parts of the country.

Impetigo is identified by the type of lesion (or sore) that appears on the skin. The following signs and symptoms usually help identify the disease.

Signs and Symptoms:
- Small red spots become tiny blisters that rupture and ooze.
- Ooze from the blister produces a sticky, honey-colored crust.
- Lesions are easily spread to other parts of the body by scratching.

In a small percentage of cases, children with impetigo develop a kidney problem called *glomerulonephritis*. This kidney condition will cause the urine to turn a dark brown. The child may also complain of a headache, and the child's blood pressure may rise.

Although the problem sounds serious, most children recover completely and quickly. Treatment with antibiotics may not prevent the kidney problem, but it can stop the spread of impetigo and prevent the disease from spreading to other children.

Suggestions for Teachers and Caregivers

✓ Observe children with skin sores or bites for signs of impetigo.

✓ If the sores can be identified as impetigo, contact the parents and check to see if they are aware of the problem. If not, discuss your observations.

✓ Practice good hygiene. Encourage children to wash their hands frequently with soap and water. Discourage scratching.

✓ Wash all toys or objects that have come into contact with the child's sores.

✓ If a child with impetigo continues to come to daycare or school with sores that are not improving, if the lesions seem to be spreading, if the child has more than one or two lesions, or if the child develops the signs of glomerulonephritis, contact the parents immediately. Encourage the parents to take the child to a physician for treatment.

✓ Children may be allowed to stay in daycare or school if they practice good personal hygiene. Children who are excluded may return when all the lesions are dry.

✓ Observe other children in the classroom for signs and symptoms of impetigo.

Ringworm

---————————— **Suggestions for Parents** ———————————

✓ If your child has impetigo, treat the condition as soon as possible to prevent the spread of the sores to other parts of the body or to other children.

✓ If the child has only one or two sores, soak them in warm water to remove the crusts. Wash the sores with soap and water and apply an over-the-counter triple antibiotic ointment. (Some medical authorities believe that soap and water are enough to treat the sores.) You can cover the sores with a clean dressing, such as a Band-Aid, to help prevent the child from spreading the infection.

✓ If the sores do not heal quickly, if they seem to be spreading, or if signs of the kidney condition glomerulonephritis occur, have your child examined by a doctor. Doctors usually prescribe an antibiotic to be taken by mouth to treat the infection.

✓ If daycare or school officials have excluded your child from attendance, the child may return when all the sores are dry.

Ringworm

Ringworm is not caused by a worm, as the name suggests, but by a fungus that creates a red, scaly ring around a clear center. The technical name for ringworm is *tinea*. When it occurs on the body, it is called *tinea corporis,* which means *ringworm of the body*. Ringworm can also occur on the scalp as *tinea capitis* and on the foot as *tinea pedis* or *athlete's foot*.

Ringworm is spread by direct contact with infected humans, animals or objects (combs, towels). The disease can be spread as long as the characteristic ringworm sores are present. Ringworm occurs more often during the warm months and in warmer climates. Good hygiene practices such as bathing, drying thoroughly with clean linens and not sharing towels or washcloths can reduce the chances of contracting ringworm.

Ringworm

Signs and Symptoms:
- Initial marks begin as small, red bumps that spread outward.
- As the bumps spread outward, the center clears, leaving a border that looks like a red, scaly outer ring.
- Sores are frequently itchy.
- With ringworm, there are no scabs, pus or crusts as in impetigo.

Suggestions for Teachers and Caregivers

✓ If a child is itching and you observe the signs and symptoms of ringworm, contact the parents to see if they are aware of the problem. If not, discuss your observations.

✓ Be sure that good handwashing techniques are practiced at the daycare center or school. Children with ringworm should wash their hands frequently with soap and water.

✓ If the child remains in school, ask parents to cover the lesions with a dressing to help prevent scratching and spreading of the infection.

✓ If no improvement occurs after a week, call the parents and suggest that they take the child to the doctor.

Suggestions for Parents

✓ If your child has the signs and symptoms of ringworm, treat the condition as soon as possible. Apply an over-the-counter medication for ringworm to the affected area. (See Appendix B for examples.) Cover the infected area and at least one-half inch around the area with the medication.

✓ If improvement in the condition does not occur within a week, consult your doctor. The child may need a prescription for an oral medication to get rid of the infection.

✓ If the child tends to scratch the sores, cover the area with a dressing to reduce the spread of the disease.

✓ Discuss good hygiene practices for washing and drying the body with your child. Wash all the child's towels and linens in hot, soapy water to prevent the spread of the fungi spores. Clean all contaminated articles such as toys and clothing with hot, soapy water.

✓ Your child may attend daycare and school, but should be taught to practice good hygiene to prevent the spread of the infection.

Conjunctivitis

Conjunctivitis or pink eye is another communicable skin infection that frequently occurs in children. Pink eye may be caused by a virus, a bacteria or an allergy. It is only contagious when it is viral or bacterial. As the name implies, pink eye causes an irritation to the outer layer of the eyeball, making it appear pink or red and irritated. The inner surface of the eyelid is also affected.

Bacterial and viral conjunctivitis are very contagious. The disease is spread to others by contact with the discharge from the eye or the mouth or nose of infected persons, as well as by contaminated fingers and contaminated objects such as washcloths or towels. Bacterial infections are very common and are usually caused by *pneumococci* or *staphylococci* bacteria. Signs and symptoms for either viral or bacterial infections are similar. They may include any or all of the following.

Signs and Symptoms:

- The sclera (the outer portion of the eyeball that covers the white of the eye) is red or pink, and the inner lining of the eyelid is inflamed. One or both eyes may be infected.
- Eyes are sensitive to light.
- Little or no itching in the eye.

Conjunctivitis

- The eye secretes a pussy discharge.
- Dried discharge may prevent the eye from opening after sleep.
- Eyelid is swollen.
- The eye produces excessive watering or tearing.

Allergic conjunctivitis, caused by allergic reactions, has many of the same signs and symptoms listed above. However, with allergic conjunctivitis, the child often has intense itching and burning of the eyes, and both eyes are usually involved.

Suggestions for Teachers and Caregivers

✓ If a child has the signs and symptoms of pink eye, contact the parents to determine if they are aware of the condition and what is being done for treatment.

✓ Since most cases of pink eye are highly contagious, encourage children to wash their hands frequently and practice good hygiene to prevent the spread of infection.

✓ Clean all articles that may be contaminated with the infection.

✓ Observe other children in the class for signs that infection is spreading.

✓ In most cases, unless the child cannot practice good hygiene to prevent the spread of the infection, she or he may continue to attend daycare or school unless prohibited by school policy.

Suggestions for Parents

✓ If your child has any of the signs and symptoms of pink eye, contact your doctor for suggestions for treatment. Most doctors prescribe an eye solution or ointment to treat bacterial infections. Follow the directions as indicated. With viral infections, no treatment may be necessary since antibiotics will not affect viral infections. Only the symptoms can be treated. For allergic conjunctivitis, treatment will not cure the condition, but may relieve some of the symptoms. For example, antihistamines may be helpful in relieving some of the itching.

✓ Teach your child good hygiene practices to avoid spreading the infection. Encourage the child to wash his or her hands frequently. Avoid sharing of towels or washcloths. Properly dispose of any tissues that may have been used to wipe the discharge from the eye.

✓ You may continue to send your child to daycare or school as long as the child is old enough to practice good hygiene and there is no other reason why the child may not attend school, such as fever or illness from another infectious disease. (Sometimes conjunctivitis occurs with measles.)

Mouth Lesions

Another common skin problem in children is mouth lesions. Mouth sores can result from bacterial or viral infections, from injury to the mouth by such acts as biting the inside of the cheek or from allergic reactions.

The most common mouth lesions are caused by the herpes virus. Herpes infections often occur with fever and are commonly known as fever blisters. The first time a child has herpes, the sores are located in the mouth, while future infections usually affect only the lips. Herpes infections begin with blisters that change to small spots with ulcerated centers surrounded by red edges. The infection is usually triggered by fever, sunlight, tension or stress. The sores are painful.

Another mouth lesion that is common in children is a canker sore. These sores usually occur after some type of injury to the mouth, such as biting the tongue or inner cheek. Usually these heal on their own very quickly, although some children continue to bite the injured area and prolong the healing process.

A third type of mouth lesion that may occur in children is mouth ulcers.

Mouth Lesions

Some children may develop mouth ulcers when they are having an allergic reaction to a drug they're taking for another disease. Parents should consult their doctor when this type of reaction seems to be occurring.

A bacterial mouth lesion that may occur in young children, although it is more common in older children and adults, is necrotizing ulcerative gingivitis or trench mouth. Trench mouth causes sores and inflammation of the gums and produces a foul-smelling mouth odor. The child will need to see a physician or dentist for treatment. The child may need an antibiotic as well as instruction on care of the teeth and gums to prevent future infections.

Any sore in the mouth that does not heal within two weeks should be examined by a physician or dentist.

Suggestions for Teachers and Caregivers

✓ When a child complains of mouth lesions, check for other symptoms. If the child has other symptoms that would exclude her or him from school, such as fever, extreme pain or body rash, call the parents to take the child home.

✓ If there is no health reason to exclude the child from school, send a note home or call the parents at the end of the day to notify them of the child's complaint.

✓ If the child has fever blisters, encourage her or him to practice good hygiene to prevent the spread of the herpes virus. These hygienic practices should include frequent handwashing and the use of disposable towels and cups.

Suggestions for Parents

✓ If your child has mouth lesions, try to identify the underlying cause of the problem.

Mouth Lesions

✓ If the mouth lesions are caused by a virus, they will heal on their own. Treatment will help relieve symptoms, but will not cure the condition. Some topical over-the-counter medications for mouth lesions will help relieve pain. (See Appendix B for examples.) Use as directed on the label.

✓ If the mouth lesions are caused by a bacterial infection, the child may need an antibiotic. A physician can determine if the infection is bacterial. Warm salt-water rinses may help control the bad breath that often occurs with bacterial infections. Salt water destroys bacteria that cause the odor.

✓ Rinse canker sores with warm salt-water to relieve the pain and help the sores to heal.

✓ Practice good hygiene to prevent the spread of the infection. Frequent handwashing and using separate towels, washcloths, cups and eating utensils may help to prevent the spread of contagious mouth lesions.

Some skin rashes and lesions are highly contagious while others are not. For rashes and lesions that are not easily spread, early treatment may prevent the child from experiencing any unnecessary pain and discomfort from the condition. For those conditions that are easily spread, the spread of the infection must also be controlled.

The role of the caregiver is to be able to recognize the skin problem quickly and follow the recommendations for treatment and control of the infection.

Chapter 4

Catchy Problems: Common Communicable Diseases

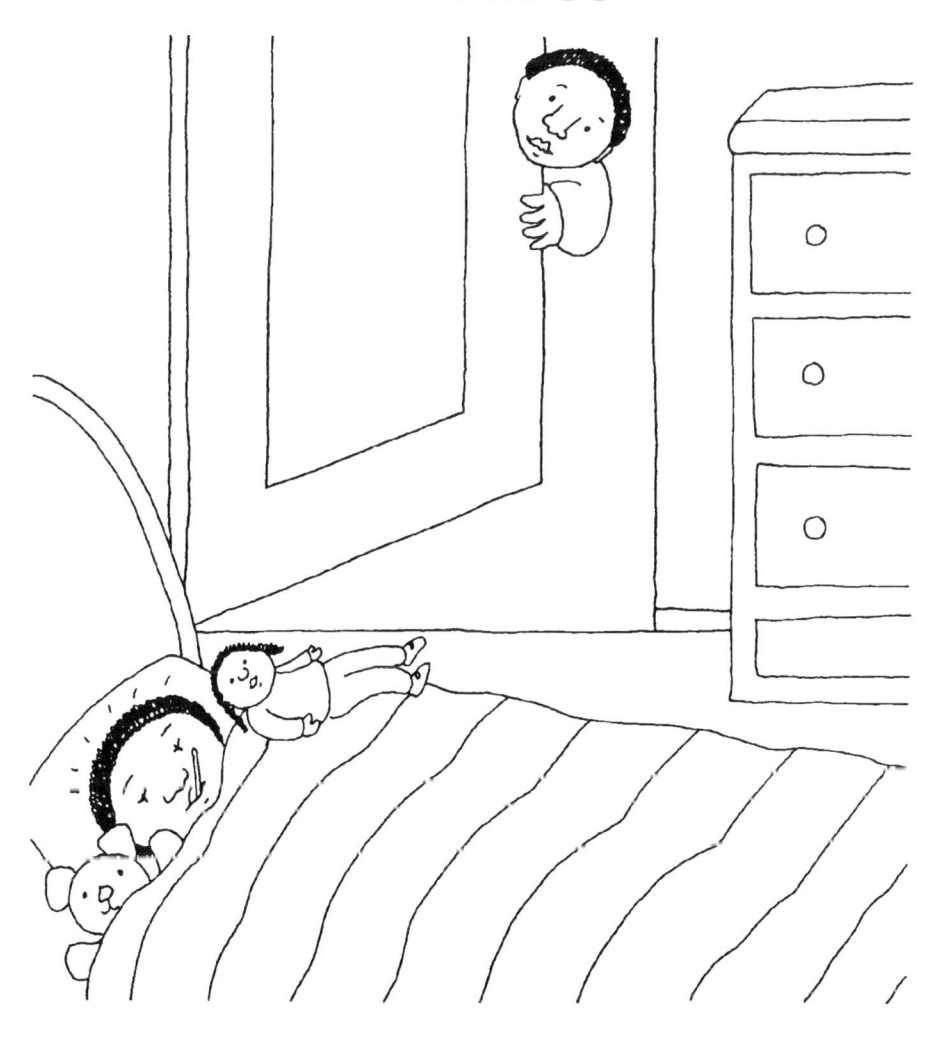

One of my wise elders, my mother, once told me that having a sick child every once in a while was part of being a parent. These words of consolation, however, didn't make me feel better when my son got sick. Like most parents, I had hoped that my child would never get sick.

Fortunately, children today do not have to experience some of the illnesses that once were common, crippling and even fatal. Medical science has developed immunizations to protect children from some of these diseases. Better sanitation and clean water have also helped to reduce illness among our children.

Frequent handwashing can prevent the spread of many communicable diseases. It is an essential habit for all children to practice. However, teachers and even parents often do not recognize and stress this habit. The importance of this single behavior—handwashing—cannot be emphasized enough!

In one of my classes in which many elementary teachers were enrolled, we were discussing the importance of handwashing. Several of the teachers remarked that they had stopped letting children wash their hands in the school bathrooms because they made such a mess. Once the teachers realized that so many infectious diseases could be prevented by simple handwashing, they developed a plan for teaching children to use the bathrooms appropriately.

Although immunizations and good hygiene protect our children against many diseases, most children still get sick. The best that we can do is to recognize the illness as soon as possible and treat the problem promptly. Early treatment can reduce the chance of complications that may result if we don't take care of the problem. Another important consideration for daycare centers and schools is preventing other children from getting the same disease.

Children may get many communicable diseases for which there are no immunizations. Many of these diseases are viral and cannot be cured with antibiotics. Parents can only treat the symptoms of such diseases. Others are bacterial, and antibiotic treatment is beneficial. The most common of these communicable diseases are chickenpox, fifth disease, the common cold and influenza.

Chickenpox

One of my college students came to school one day covered with what I thought was acne. He came by to tell me he had been out with chickenpox. This common communicable disease is usually contracted during the early childhood years, but it can occur at any age. Chickenpox is so common that almost all children catch it at some point.

Chickenpox is a highly contagious virus that causes fever and a rash. The rash will form small raised bumps that turn into blisters and often itch. The disease is easily transmitted from person to person by direct contact, droplets or airborne secretions of an infected person. Chickenpox may be transmitted as long as five days but usually one to two days before the rash appears to not more than six days after the last rash has occurred. Usually when all the scabs have crusted over, the child is not infectious.

Some children with chickenpox are very ill, while others are only mildly affected. Some children are covered in blisters, while others only have small patches. Some have a hard time with the itching, while others don't seem to be bothered.

My cousin's three children all had chickenpox at the same time. One child was very sick, while the other two were only mildly affected. Although they were all covered with the rash, the amount of itching also varied with each child.

Two problems are associated with severe itching of chickenpox—infection of the sores and scarring of the skin. These problems are caused by children scratching the blisters.

I Don't Feel Good

Chickenpox

Signs and Symptoms:

- The day before the rash appears, the child may be tired, run a slight fever and complain of a headache.
- The rash usually first appears on the back and neck and then spreads to the face and limbs. The flat red rash becomes raised, looking somewhat like insect bites, and then develops into small blisters.
- When the tiny blisters, called vesicles, break, the sores crust over. The sores are usually very itchy and are easily broken when scratched. New sores appear in stages for two to six days.
- While the child is breaking out with the vesicles, she or he may run a fever. After all the crusts have formed, the fever usually goes away.

――― *Suggestions for Teachers and Caregivers* ―――

✓ If a child has the signs and symptoms of chickenpox, call the parents to come get the child and take her or him home.

✓ All people in contact with the child should wash their hands with soap and water.

✓ If anyone in the class has a condition such as leukemia, Hodgkin's disease or AIDS that causes him or her to be in serious danger and at risk for any infections, his or her parents should be notified. A substance called Varicella Zoster Immune Globulin (VZIG) can be given within 72 hours of exposure to prevent disease.

✓ The infected child may return to school when all the sores have crusted over and no new blisters are present, usually a minimum of seven days after the rash.

――― *Suggestions for Parents* ―――

✓ If your child has the signs and symptoms of chickenpox, keep him or her away from other people until all the blisters have crusted over.

✓ To help reduce the fever and to make the child more comfortable, many physicians recommend acetaminophen. ***Do not give aspirin to a child with chickenpox*** because of the possibility of contracting Reye's syndrome.

✓ Warm baths with baking soda (1/2 cup soda for each tub of water) may help reduce the itching. Calamine lotion can also be used to relieve the itching. If the itching is severe, the doctor may prescribe an antihistamine. Cutting the child's fingernails and having the child wear gloves can reduce the chances of scarring from scratching.

✓ Keep the hands and skin clean. Handwashing is very important to prevent the spread of the infection or bacterial infections that may occur from scratching.

✓ The child may return to school a minimum of seven days after the rash has appeared and when all the blisters have crusted over.

Fifth Disease

Fifth disease got its name because it is the fifth of the five most common rashes that used to affect children. The rashes were chickenpox, measles, rubella, roseola and fifth disease. Today with immunizations for measles and rubella, fifth disease is really misnamed.

The disease is caused by a virus, specifically parvovirus B19. Because the rash caused by fifth disease is so similar to other rashes, many children are excluded from school unnecessarily. Fifth disease is highly communicable but relatively harmless in children. Severe complications from the virus are unusual. There is no treatment for the disease.

Signs and Symptoms:

- For most children, the only symptom is a light red rash on the face. Children look as if they have been slapped on the cheeks. As the

disease progresses, the rash may be found on the backs of the arms and legs and tends to come and go.
- The rash on the face usually fades in four days and is gone on the rest of the body in seven days, although it may recur for days or weeks.

Suggestions for Teachers and Caregivers

✓ If you recognize the possible symptoms of fifth disease, notify the parents of your suspicions. Children do not have to be excluded from daycare or school.

Suggestions for Parents

✓ If you suspect fifth disease, watch the child to be sure that this disease is the problem. Check the child for fever. There is usually no fever with fifth disease. If there is fever, you should consider the other possible problems and courses of action suggested in this book.

✓ You may send your child to daycare or school. There are no restrictions on activities.

The Common Cold

The name *common cold* was given to this upper respiratory infection because almost all people at some time will have a cold. It is probably the most common communicable disease that children experience.

The illness usually lasts about seven days. It is transmitted by direct contact or by airborne droplets. Most colds are spread by just touching an infected person. Washing hands frequently while you are around an infected person can greatly reduce the chances that you will get the cold.

The Common Cold

The common cold is caused by more than ninety different viruses, so treatment mainly consists of treating the symptoms. Complications from colds may lead to bacterial infections, such as ear infections, sinus infections and bronchitis. The cold may be spread to others one day before symptoms appear to five days afterward.

Signs and Symptoms:

- The most common signs and symptoms are a runny nose, watery eyes, irritability, scratchy throat and complaints of being tired.
- Children may also complain that they can't breathe through the nose.

Suggestions for Teachers and Caregivers

✓ A child with a cold may continue to go to daycare or school unless the child develops other symptoms that would indicate the need to exclude him or her from school, such as fever or excessive coughing.

✓ Practice good hygiene. Everyone should wash his or her hands frequently to prevent the spread of disease. A child with a cold should carefully dispose of any dirty tissues that she or he has used. All children should be taught to cover their mouths and noses when coughing or sneezing.

✓ Limit activities that may cause infected children to have more difficulty breathing, such as running, vigorous physical education activities or dancing.

Suggestions for Parents

✓ Teach your child to cover his or her mouth and nose when coughing or sneezing.

✓ The child may also need to be taught how to blow her or his nose.

The Common Cold

Excessive blowing can cause the infection to be forced into the tube that goes to the ear and could lead to a middle ear infection. The proper way to blow your nose is to blow softly through one nostril and then the other. (Do not cover one nostril while blowing the other; this practice creates excessive pressure in the nostril through which you are blowing.)

✓ Carefully dispose of any tissues that are soiled with the cold discharges.

✓ Wash hands frequently to prevent the spread of the disease.

✓ Encourage the child to drink plenty of fluids. Don't worry if the child is not hungry, but do get him or her to drink liquids.

✓ For stuffed-up noses, salt-water nosedrops can help breathing. Mix 1/2 teaspoon of **non-iodized** salt with one cup of water. Be sure to use **non-iodized** salt. Iodized salt will cause a burning feeling in the nasal tissues. Tilt the child's head back, and drop several drops in each nostril. You can also buy saline nose drops over-the-counter at your local drugstore. Try not to use over-the-counter medicated nose drops. They may be habit forming, and they can cause harmful side effects when overused. Medicated nose drops, even those designed for children, should never be used for more than three days.

✓ Use a cool-mist humidifier at night to provide moisture in the air while the child is sleeping. The moisture will help the child breathe easier.

✓ Depending upon the age of your child, some over-the-counter medications may be helpful. Antihistamines will stop the runny nose, and decongestants will help open the nasal passages for breathing. Consult your pharmacist for recommendations and follow the directions on the container.

✓ If the child is tired, encourage her or him to rest. Determine the allowed activity level by how the child feels.

✓ Your child may continue to go to daycare or school as long as he or she feels well enough and does not have any symptoms that would interfere with performance, such as excessive coughing or fever.

Influenza

Influenza is a more serious viral infection that frequently affects young children. Commonly called the *flu,* influenza is an infectious disease of the respiratory tract. It is spread by direct contact with airborne droplets or by nose or throat discharges from an infected person. Influenza can last up to seven days and occasionally longer.

Signs and Symptoms:

- Influenza usually starts with a sudden onset of fever. Fever is followed by a severe cough, chills, headache and general achiness.

―――― *Suggestions for Teachers and Caregivers* ――――

✓ Since influenza is highly contagious, children with the signs and symptoms should be sent home. Call the parents to come get the child as soon as possible.

✓ Encourage all children and staff to wash their hands frequently to prevent the spread of infection.

✓ Call the local health department if there is a significant increase in absences due to influenza.

✓ Exclude all infected children and staff until their symptoms are gone.

―――― *Suggestions for Parents* ――――

✓ For fever, headache and the general achiness associated with influenza, doctors may recommend acetaminophen. ***Do not give aspirin to a child with influenza*** because it may lead to complications including Reye's syndrome.

✓ A cool-mist humidifier may help relieve coughing.

I Don't Feel Good

Influenza

✓ Gargling with salt water can help relieve the pain of sore throat. Mix one teaspoon of salt in one cup of warm water for gargling.

✓ Encourage the child to drink plenty of fluids.

✓ If the child develops rapid breathing, ear pain, a severe sore throat or symptoms that last more than seven days, call your doctor or make an appointment to have your child examined.

✓ Physical exertion should be discouraged while the symptoms persist.

✓ The child should not return to daycare or school until all the symptoms are gone.

We may not be able to prevent children from getting sick all the time, but with just a little bit of information, we can make sure that sick children get well quickly and have as few complications as possible!

Chapter 5

Preventing Problems: Immunizable Diseases

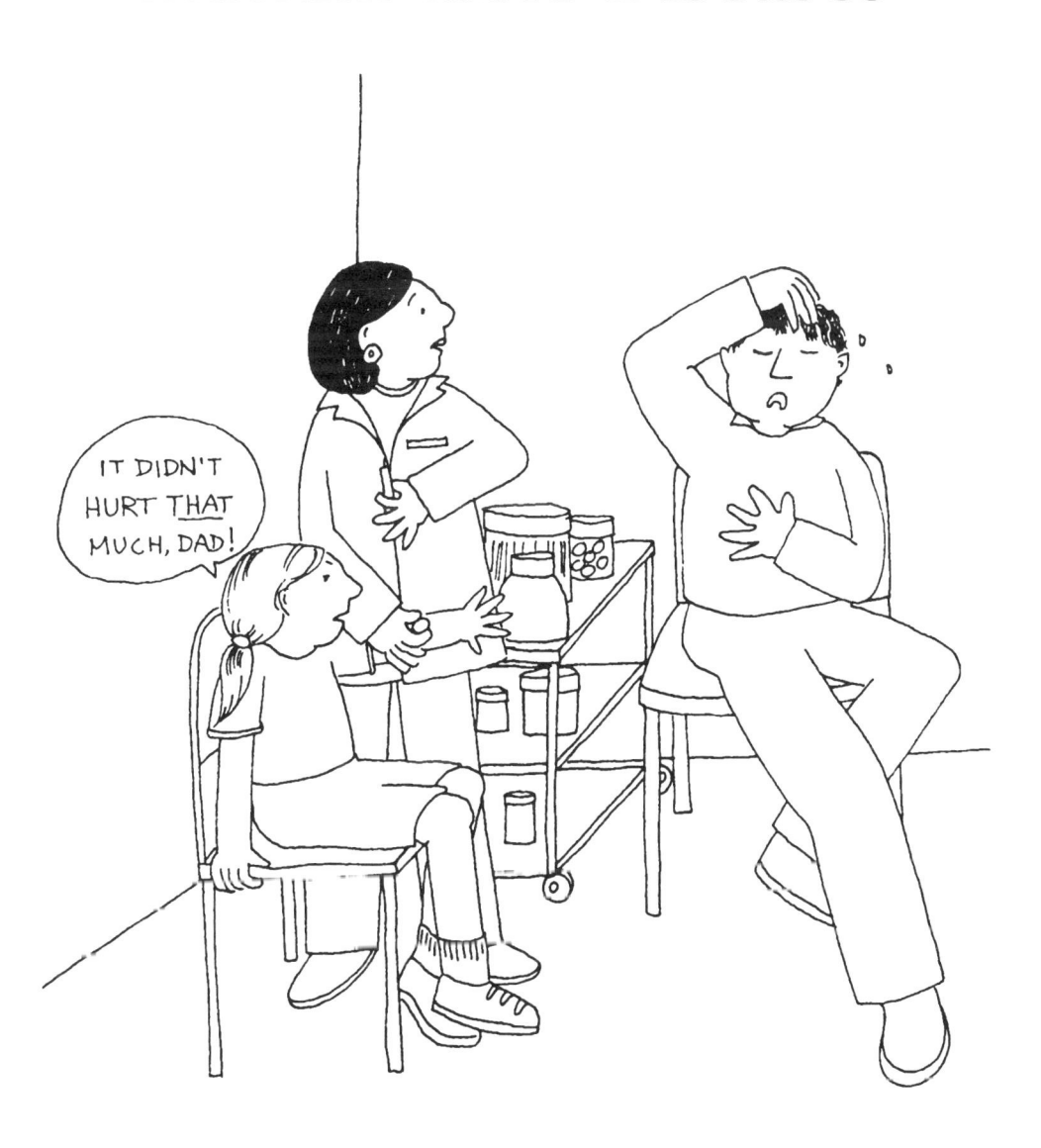

What are immunizable diseases? Simply, immunizable diseases are diseases that can be prevented by taking a special shot or a pill. A vaccine is a substance that is taken orally or by injection. In a reaction to the vaccine, the body manufactures its own defenses. Then the body can fight future exposures to the disease. Thanks to immunizations, children no longer have to experience such diseases as smallpox, polio, diptheria, pertussis (whooping cough), tetanus, mumps, measles and rubella.

However, immunizations can protect children from disease only if they are given as recommended. Before children enter daycare or school, they should have begun receiving immunizations that will protect them from disease. Appendix D lists the recommended immunizations and their schedules according to the American Academy of Pediatrics.

As recommended by the American Academy of Pediatrics, by the time children are in kindergarten, most of their immunizations should be completed. In many states, children are not allowed to enroll in school until their immunizations are up-to-date. Many local health departments report an increase in September every year in the number of school-age children who come to immunization clinics to get their immunizations so they can remain in school.

The big question that many people in the health professions ask about immunizations is, Why aren't all children immunized as soon as possible and especially before they go to school? We know that doctors encourage all new parents to get their children immunized, but research indicates that fewer parents are doing so.

Many new parents have not seen and are not aware of the disabilities and complications of the immunizable diseases. Some parents may think that because the diseases are so rare they just don't occur anymore. These parents are wrong! Children still get these diseases. Many children are needlessly suffering from complications of these diseases because they were not immunized.

One of the serious immunizable diseases that has recurred in many areas of the United States is measles. Some of the children who have measles have not been vaccinated. Others were vaccinated, but the type of vaccine that was used was not effective. Another group contracting measles are children who received the vaccination before they were fifteen months old. Such an early measles vaccination is not as successful as vaccination of children older than 15 months.

Because of the recent measles epidemics in this country, the American Academy of Pediatrics has recommended that all children who received a measles vaccination prior to 15 months of age be revaccinated. A second measles vaccination (MMR) is also recommended for children at entry to middle or junior high school. Some institutions of higher education are also requiring proof of two vaccinations for measles and rubella before entry into college, as recommended by the Centers for Disease Control and the American College Health Association.

All the recommended immunizations can be obtained from your family doctor, pediatrician or public health department. Fees will vary according to where you go for the immunization, although the serum comes from the same source. Usually, the health department is the least expensive place to get immunizations, but it gives the immunizations only on certain days of the week. Where to get the immunizations is a matter of parental preference.

Although the immunizable diseases except measles are rarely seen, all parents, teachers and caregivers should be aware of the signs and symptoms and know what to do in case a child contracts such a disease.

Diptheria

One of the first immunizations that is given to a child is the DTP immunization. The child is immunized for three diseases—diptheria, tetanus and pertussis—in one shot.

Diptheria is an infectious bacterial disease that affects the nose, throat and skin. It is transmitted from person to person by airborne droplets.

Diptheria

Complications include paralysis and heart damage. About 5 to 10 percent of those contracting diptheria die.

Signs and Symptoms:
- Enlarged lymph nodes may be found in the neck.
- The child will usually have a sore throat with patches of grayish membrane in the nose or throat.

―――― *Suggestions for Teachers and Caregivers* ――――

✓ Encourage parents to take the child to a physician if the child has signs or symptoms of diptheria.

✓ If a child has diptheria, parents should notify the school so children and staff can be observed for sore throats for seven days.

✓ A child with diptheria should be excluded from school until he or she has two negative cultures taken not less than 24 hours apart and not less than 24 hours after antibiotic treatment is finished.

✓ In confirmed cases, the school is required to report the disease to the local health department.

―――――― *Suggestions for Parents* ――――――

✓ Have your child immunized for diptheria as recommended by the American Academy of Pediatrics.

✓ If your child has the signs and symptoms of diptheria, take him or her to a physician for diagnosis and treatment.

✓ Follow recommended antibiotic treatment and quarantine procedures as described by your physician. (Such procedures may include isolating your child from others until two negative cultures have been obtained or for at least fourteen days.)

✓ Disinfect all articles that have been in contact with the child.

✓ Have a doctor do a throat and nose culture of all intimate contacts (siblings, parents, best friends, etc.) to check for presence of the bacteria that causes diptheria. If these people have not been immunized against diptheria, they should be immunized immediately.

✓ Notify school officials so they can observe other children and staff.

Tetanus

Tetanus, commonly called lockjaw, is caused by the tetanus bacteria. The bacteria are present in dust, soil and human or animal wastes. Since the tetanus germ grows in places that are not exposed to air, injuries that are caused by sharp objects or punctures are the wounds that are likely to introduce the bacteria into the body. This is why people associate the spread of the disease with stepping on a rusty nail. Without the protection provided by the tetanus immunization, death can occur in 35 to 70 percent of the people who contract the disease.

Even if one recovers, tetanus is a very painful disease. Several years ago when I visited in India and studied health systems, I saw a woman recovering from tetanus. Like many women who have not been immunized, she had contracted tetanus during childbirth. She was still rigid from the waist up, with all the muscles in her face contracting at the same time.

I understood then why the disease is called lockjaw. Seeing that woman made me appreciate the availability of immunizations in the United States. I would hate to see any of my family, especially my child, experience that most painful disease.

I Don't Feel Good

Signs and Symptoms:

- Tetanus causes painful muscular contractions, often in the neck and jaw area.
- A common first sign is rigid abdominal muscles.

———— Suggestions for Teachers and Caregivers ————

✓ If you suspect that a child has a sharp puncture injury, notify the parents. Suggest that they check to see if the child's tetanus immunization is up-to-date. If it isn't, parents should be encouraged to take their child to the doctor for a tetanus booster shot.

✓ Since tetanus is not a communicable disease, there are no recommendations for exclusion from school.

———— Suggestions for Parents ————

✓ Have your child immunized for tetanus as recommended by the American Academy of Pediatrics.

✓ If your child has incurred a puncture wound or cut, such as a wound caused by a rusty nail, and the child has not had a tetanus shot within the past five years, take him or her to a doctor for a tetanus booster shot. (Tetanus bacteria grow best in wounds where there is no air. If you are unsure about the wound, call your doctor for advice.)

✓ If your child develops signs and symptoms of tetanus, seek immediate medical treatment.

Pertussis

Pertussis is a highly contagious bacterial infection commonly known as whooping cough, because of the characteristic whooping sound made when the child breathes in during a prolonged coughing bout. Infants who contract the disease often die, but death is rare for children over the age of two. The disease can be spread through airborne droplets and direct contact with an infected person.

Signs and Symptoms:

- Stage One—For one to three weeks, the child may have coughing, sneezing, a runny nose and occasional vomiting.
- Stage Two—The child has continuous coughing with characteristic whooping sound accompanied by sweating, exhaustion, vomiting an excessive amount of thick mucus lasting for two to four weeks.
- Recovery Stage—The coughing gradually stops in two to three weeks.

Suggestions for Teachers and Caregivers

✓ If you suspect a child has pertussis, encourage the parents to take the child to the physician.

✓ In confirmed cases, notify the local health department.

✓ A child with pertussis who is on antibiotic treatment may return to school after five days. If not on antibiotic treatment, the child should be excluded from school until four weeks after the onset of the illness or until the cough has stopped.

✓ Observe other children and staff for signs and symptoms of pertussis, and encourage parents to seek immediate treatment if necessary.

✓ All close contacts under the age of three, even if they have been immunized, should receive antibiotic treatment for ten days after the infected child has been excluded from school.

✓ Contacts under the age of seven years of age who have been immunized should receive a booster dose of pertussis unless one has been given in the last six months.

I Don't Feel Good

Polio

———————— *Suggestions for Parents* ————————

✓ Have your child immunized for pertussis as recommended by the American Academy of Pediatrics.

✓ If you suspect your child has pertussis, take her or him to a doctor for diagnosis and treatment.

✓ If your child has pertussis, follow doctor's orders for antibiotic treatment.

✓ Your child may return to school after five days of antibiotic therapy. If no antibiotics are taken, your child may need to be excluded from school for at least four weeks or until the coughing has stopped.

✓ Be sure to notify school officials, so they can observe other children and staff for signs and symptoms.

✓ Close family contacts should be on antibiotic treatment for the duration of the infected child's cough.

Polio

Polio is an infectious viral disease that can have minor or more serious effects. The serious effects include paralysis, meningitis and respiratory infections. The virus attacks the central nervous system. It may cause paralysis, depending on the location of the nerve cell destruction in the brain stem or the spinal cord. Polio is spread through throat discharges and feces. The best way to prevent polio is through the oral polio virus immunization.

Signs and Symptoms:

- Some of the common signs of polio are fever, headache, gastrointestinal disturbances and discomfort and stiffness of the neck and back.
- In some cases, paralysis may also occur.

──────── *Suggestions for Teachers and Caregivers* ────────

✓ Report signs and symptoms to the parents and suggest that the child be seen by a physician.

✓ If the child is confirmed to have polio, notify the local health department.

✓ Check the immunization records for all children in the school. Strongly encourage the parents of those children without up-to-date polio immunization to begin the immunizations.

──────── *Suggestions for Parents* ────────

✓ Have your child immunized for polio as recommended by the American Academy of Pediatrics.

✓ If your child has the signs and symptoms of polio, seek medical advice. The signs and symptoms listed above for polio can also indicate other diseases such as meningitis, infectious mononucleosis or paralysis caused by a tick bite.

✓ Follow the instructions from your physician for care and treatment. (Since polio is so rare, specific suggestions are not listed.)

Measles

Measles, or rubeola, is a highly contagious viral illness that used to be very common in childhood. Finally, in 1966, an adequate vaccination was developed for measles. Measles is spread by nasal droplets or direct contact with nasal or throat secretions of an infected person. A child remains contagious from four days before the rash appears until four days after the appearance of the rash.

Measles

Children should receive two doses of the measles vaccine. The first immunization should be given at fifteen months or as soon as possible thereafter. The second dose, designed to boost measles and mumps immunity, should be given to children 11-12 years or older who have not had measles. According to the American Academy of Pediatrics, if mealses outbreaks occur in the community, the MMR booster may be given at entry to kindergarten or at an earlier age. Both doses should be given as the combined measles, mumps and rubella vaccine.

Signs and Symptoms:

- When measles begins, the child may have fever, weakness, dry cough, runny nose and red, irritated eyes that are sensitive to light.
- In three to five days, fine white spots on a red base appear inside the mouth near the cheek. (These are called Koplik spots.)
- About the fifth day, the Koplik spots fade and a rash appears around the hairline and on the face and neck and behind the ears. As the spots mature, large red patches form. The rash then spreads from the head and neck to the chest, abdomen and finally, the arms and legs. By the time the rash is on the arms and legs, the rash on the head is fading. The rash lasts from four to seven days and may itch.

―――― *Suggestions for Teachers and Caregivers* ――――

✓ If you suspect a child may have measles, contact the parents and suggest that they take the child to a doctor. Since measles is a highly contagious disease, confirmed cases must be reported to the local health department.

✓ Check immunization records of the children and staff at the school to be sure they are protected with the measles vaccination. If any children have not been inoculated, encourage their parents to have them immunized as soon as possible, or exclude the children until they show proof of immunization after fifteen months of age.

✓ A child with measles should not be allowed to return to school until at least five days after the rash begins.

---------- *Suggestions for Parents* ----------

✓ Have your child immunized for measles as recommended by the American Academy of Pediatrics.

✓ If your child has the signs and symptoms of measles, contact your physician. The physician should report any confirmed cases of measles to the local health department.

✓ If the child is diagnosed with measles, she or he will need to be isolated while contagious. Do not send the child back to school until at least five days after the rash appears.

✓ Since the child may be sensitive to light, you may need to dim the light in the child's room to make him or her more comfortable. Some physicians recommend that acetaminophen be given to reduce the fever. **Remember, do not give aspirin to a child.** A humidifier may also be used if the child has a cough.

✓ If the child develops any of the following signs or symptoms, **call the doctor immediately:**
    severe headache, vomiting or convulsions
    bleeding from the nose, mouth or rectum or unusual bruising
    difficulty breathing

✓ You should also take your child to the doctor if she or he develops an earache, sore throat or rapid breathing.

✓ If you have any other children in your family who are not immunized, have them immunized for measles immediately.

Mumps

Mumps, the second M of the MMR vaccinations, is another childhood illness from which children can be protected. Mumps is a viral infection that affects the parotid and salivary glands located just above the back angle of the jaw and under the tongue. However, some people have mumps without any swelling of these glands. The disease is spread by droplets from an infected person, and a person with mumps is contagious from two days before the first symptoms to about a week after the swelling has begun. Complications very rarely occur in children.

Signs and Symptoms:

- During the first 24 hours, the child may develop a low fever and complain of a headache, earache, loss of appetite and tiredness.
- By the second day, the earache is worse when the child tries to chew or swallow. If you feed the child sour foods, such as a lemon or a dill pickle, the pain may get worse.
- On the third day, the parotid and salivary glands on one or both sides of the face usually swell, and the child complains of pain and tenderness. Fever may be high in some children, while others have only low fever.

Suggestions for Teachers and Caregivers

✓ A child with the symptoms of mumps should be checked by a physician. Contact the parents and have them take the child out of daycare or school. Suggest that parents take the child to the doctor. If mumps is confirmed, the school must report the case to the local health department.

✓ The child will need to be excluded from daycare or school while ill. The child may return to school a minimum of nine days after the start of swelling.

✓ Observe the other children and staff for signs of infection. Check the immunization records, and encourage all parents of children who are not protected to get them immunized.

---------- **Suggestions for Parents** ----------

✓ Have your child immunized for mumps as recommended by the American Academy of Pediatrics.

✓ If your child has the signs and symptoms of mumps, take him or her to your physician for diagnosis. The doctor will want to look for the presence of any complications, such as encephalitis (a viral infection of the brain), deafness or problems in the testes or ovaries (such complications could cause sterility).

✓ If your child has mumps, you will need to isolate her or him from other people until at least a week after the swelling in the glands has begun. You may send the child back to school nine days after the swelling first occurs.

✓ To make the child more comfortable, your physician might recommend acetaminophen for pain relief. Avoid sour foods like dill pickles and lemons or fluids such as orange juice and lemonade that could cause the child pain.

✓ Immunize other members of the family who are not protected.

Rubella

Rubella, the target of the third vaccination in the MMR immunization, is a mild viral infection. The disease is also called German measles or the three-day measles because of its short duration. Rubella is spread by droplets from the nose or mouth of an infected person. Some people may have rubella and not have any symptoms while they spread the disease to

Rubella

others. The disease can be spread seven days before the rash appears to at least four days after the rash appears.

During the first three months of pregnancy, rubella may cause serious problems for the unborn child of more than 50 percent of the women who have not had the disease or been immunized against it. The risk reduces as the pregnancy continues. Complications may include heart disease, deafness or mental retardation. Obviously, it is of utmost importance for women who may become pregnant to be protected from rubella.

Signs and Symptoms:

- Several days before the rash appears, the child may be tired and complain of a headache or have a cough, runny nose, scratchy throat and tender, swollen lymph glands at the back of the neck.
- A rash that is faint pink in color appears on the face and rapidly spreads downward. In some cases, there is no rash. The rash is usually gone by the third day.
- If the child has fever, it is usually low and only lasts for two days. Some older children experience joint pain on the third day of the illness.

―――― *Suggestions for Teachers and Caregivers* ――――

✓ Contact the parents if you suspect rubella, so they can take the child home as soon as possible. Suggest that parents take the child to the physician for diagnosis.

✓ If the child has a confirmed case of rubella, the school should notify the local health department.

✓ As with other immunizable diseases, check the records of the children and staff at the school to be sure everyone is up-to-date on immunizations. Encourage all parents to have their children immunized.

✓ The child may return to school a minimum of four days after the rash first appears.

Suggestions for Parents

✓ If your child has the signs and symptoms of rubella, contact your physician for diagnosis and treatment.

✓ If the child has a confirmed case of rubella, contact school officials, so they can notify the local health department and observe other children and staff for symptoms.

✓ Keep the child comfortable. With low fever, acetaminophen may be helpful in combating pain.

✓ Avoid exposing any pregnant woman to the child. If a pregnant woman has been exposed and she is not protected against rubella, she should be notified of the problem and counseled by her physician.

✓ You may send your child back to school on the fifth day after the rash first occurred.

✓ Check the immunization records for all the members of your family and have any unprotected person immunized.

Haemophilus Influenza Type B (HIB)

A vaccine for haemophilus influenza type B (HIB) has been available only since 1985. This vaccine is the most recent immunization recommended by the American Academy of Pediatrics. HIB is a bacteria that can cause serious illnesses such as meningitis and arthritis in children. This vaccination has reduced the leading cause of meningitis in children. It is recommended for children between two months and six years old.

Caring for children sometimes involves taking the child to the doctor or health clinic for preventive care. If you asked most pediatricians, they would prefer to see children while they were healthy and help parents maintain their children's health. However, many parents only bring their children to the doctor when they become sick. Some children become sick because they do not have the proper protection from some diseases.

A major responsibility of parents is to ensure that their children are immunized against the preventable diseases as recommended by the American Academy of Pediatrics. Schools and daycare centers can further encourage the immunizations of children by requiring that all children who attend the center or school be immunized at the earliest recommended times. If the community works together to encourage immunizations, children will be more likely to survive their childhood years with good health.

Chapter 6

Less Common Problems: Chronic Diseases

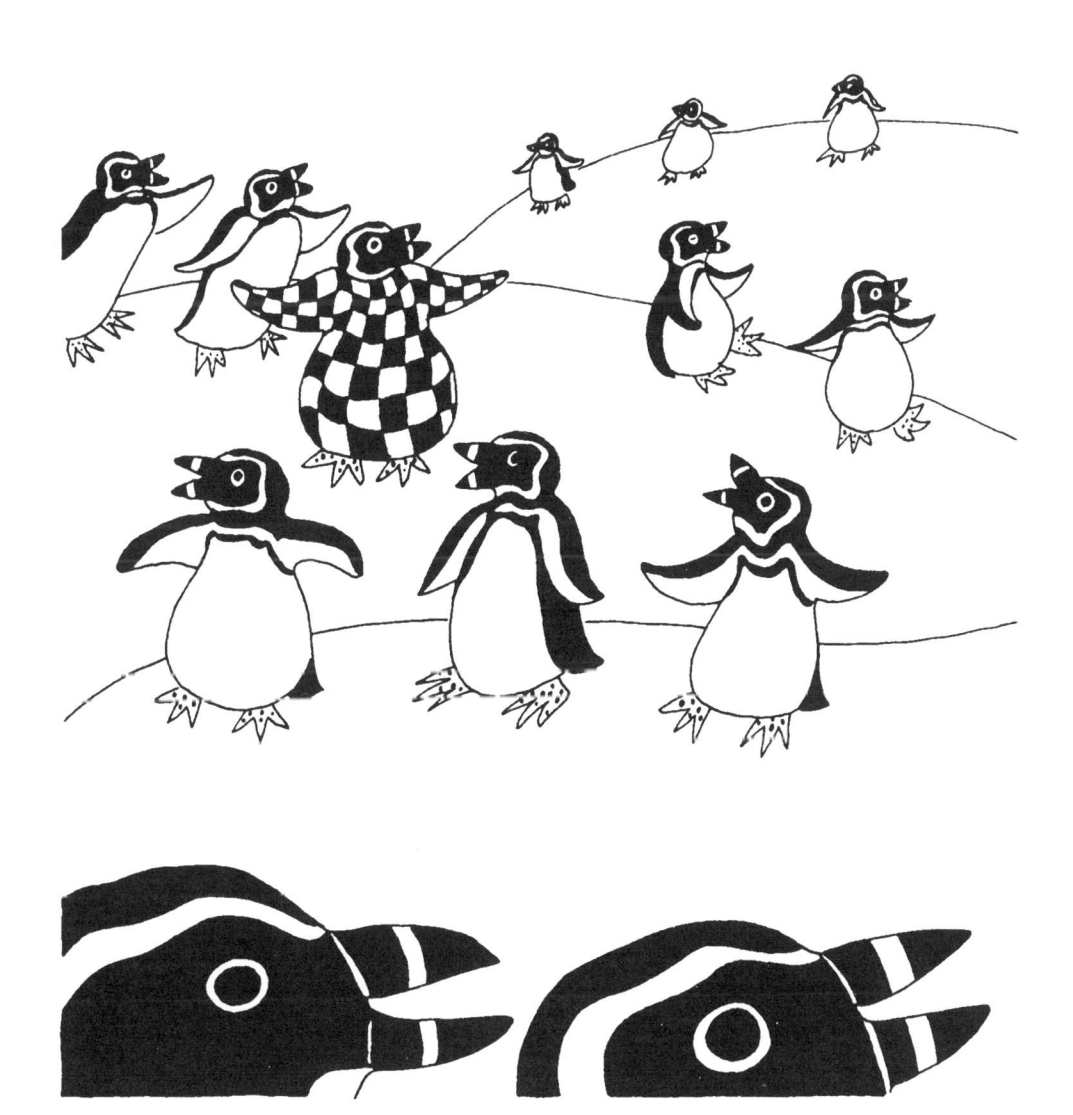

A few children will experience some less common diseases or conditions during their childhood years. These diseases and conditions are termed *chronic diseases* because they affect the child for a long time. Children with a chronic disease may not get well. They may experience disability and, in some cases, they may even die. Why one child gets sick with a chronic disease and another doesn't is usually unknown.

For children four to ten years old, chronic diseases are different from communicable diseases in several ways. First, chronic diseases are not nearly as common among children as are the communicable diseases. Second, chronic diseases are not spread from one person to another. A child with a chronic disease such as cancer cannot give it to another child. Third, a chronic disease will probably have been identified before the child starts school. (Chronic diseases sometimes develop at puberty, when hormonal changes may contribute to their onset.)

The most common chronic diseases that affect children are arthritis, cancer, diabetes, epilepsy and heart conditions. Signs and symptoms of these diseases will be presented in this chapter. Another chronic disease, AIDS, although not common in four- to ten-year-old children, will also be described. Addresses and toll-free numbers of the major voluntary organizations devoted to fighting each disease are also provided. You may contact these organizations for further information.

Arthritis

The term *arthritis* describes a collection of more than 100 different conditions known as rheumatic diseases. All of these conditions affect the joints and tissues surrounding the joints. Although the name arthritis means *inflammation of the joint,* the joint may not be inflamed in many kinds of arthritis. Arthritis should be thought of as a condition that causes problems with joints.

Juvenile rheumatoid arthritis (JRA) is the most common form of arthritis that affects children. Within this category, there are three major types of arthritis.

Systemic JRA affects the entire body. Symptoms include a very high fever, a rash and many swollen joints. The internal organs as well as the joints are affected, and the child may also have inflammation of the outer lining of the heart, stomach pain, severe anemia and a high level of white cells in the blood.

Polyarticular JRA affects five or more joints. This is the form of arthritis seen in almost half of the children with JRA. The disease usually affects the small joints of the fingers and hands, but it can also affect the weight-bearing joints. Other signs and symptoms include low fever; a positive blood test for rheumatoid factor; and lumps, called rheumatoid nodules, on parts of the body such as the elbow that receive pressure from shoes, chairs or other objects.

Pauciarticular (meaning *few joints*) JRA begins in four or fewer joints and most commonly affects large joints such as the elbows, knees or ankles. With this type of JRA, eye inflammation frequently develops and can cause blindness if not treated. Pauciarticular JRA is the second most common form of JRA. It affects 30 to 40 percent of the children with the disease.

The major signs and symptoms of any form of arthritis in children include chronic joint inflammation and pain involving one or more joints, including the fingers, wrists, elbows, hips, knees and feet. The disease may also interfere with normal growth, causing a child to be small and to walk with a stiff gait or take shorter steps.

Sometimes the signs of arthritis may not be apparent, although damage and pain are occurring inside the child's body. Sometimes the swollen joints can only be seen when the disease has caused deformities in the joints. Adults who care for children should be aware of subtle signs of the disease, such as stiffness, difficulty performing certain tasks, walking slowly and being clumsy or irritable. Many children with arthritis try so hard to be like other children that they try to ignore or conceal their stiffness and pain.

For information about childhood arthritis and suggestions for care and treatment, contact the Arthritis Foundation in your state or write the national organization.

Arthritis Foundation National Office
1314 Spring St. NW
Atlanta, GA 30309
1-800-283-7800

Cancer

The term *cancer* actually describes a variety of diseases that affect the body. Cancer refers to disorderly and uncontrolled growth of cells of the body. Cancer in children is rare, even though it is the chief cause of death from disease in children ages four to ten.

The common cancer warning signs for children are nausea, weight loss, swelling, double vision, stumbling, nosebleeds, drowsiness and listlessness. Seek medical advice for any abnormal signs and symptoms for which there is no obvious cause.

Cancers that occur in children do tend to grow more quickly than in adults. The child's body tissues are growing rapidly, and the cancer grows right along with them. The most common forms of cancer that affect children are cancers of the blood, bone, brain, nervous system and kidney.

Leukemia, the most frequent form of cancer in children, is a cancer of the blood-forming tissues. White blood cells, which usually protect the body from disease, are not able to function properly, and the child gets sick or bleeds easily.

Cancers of the nervous system are the second most frequent form of cancer in children. These cancers are known as neuroblastomas. They are commonly found in the adrenal glands located above the kidneys.

Osteogenic sarcoma is a bone cancer that usually develops in the forearm or the lower leg, although it can occur anywhere in the body.

When it occurs in an arm or leg, the limb swells, and the child may have difficulty using the arm or leg.

Brain tumors usually cause symptoms very early in the disease. Major symptoms include blurred or double vision, dizziness, difficulty in walking or handling objects and unexplained nausea.

Lymphomas are cancers that involve the lymph nodes. Lymph nodes are the body's way of protecting itself from the spread of infection. Lymphomas may cause swelling of the lymph nodes in the neck, armpit and groin. They are often accompanied by general weakness and sometimes fever.

Eye tumors usually occur in children under the age of five. The tumors first cause squinting and then a pearly spot, which may be noticed on the pupil.

Wilms tumors, cancer of the kidney, are tumors that develop in the kidneys (the pair of organs that filters waste products from the blood). The tumor usually causes a swelling or lump in the child's abdomen.

For more information about childhood cancers, contact your local office of the American Cancer Society or write the national organization.

American Cancer Society National Office
1599 Clifton Rd. NE
Atlanta, GA 30329
1-800-255-2352

Diabetes

Diabetes is a condition in which the body cannot use food in a normal way because the pancreas does not produce enough insulin. Insulin is a hormone secreted by the pancreas to help convert sugar, starches and other food into the energy the body needs to live. Without insulin, high levels of sugar build up in the blood, and damage is done to nearly every tissue in the body. The most common complications of untreated diabetes are heart disease, kidney disease, blindness, nerve damage and amputations of the limbs due to the occurrence of gangrene.

Signs and symptoms of undetected diabetes in children include frequent urination accompanied by unusual thirst, extreme hunger, rapid weight loss with easy tiring, weakness, fatigue, irritability, nausea and vomiting. Since the signs and symptoms often mimic flu, adults who care for children should be aware of the symptoms of diabetes so that the proper diagnosis may be made quickly.

One mother first suspected that her son had diabetes when she noticed that he was going to the bathroom frequently in the middle of the night. When she cleaned the toilet, she noticed that the urine spots around the toilet were thick and smelled like pancake syrup. Since there was a history of diabetes in her family, she immediately took her son to the doctor. His blood sugar was extremely high, and he was identified as a child with diabetes.

Diabetes can often be held in check by diet, exercise and insulin taken orally or injected. Most children being treated for diabetes will be taught how to manage their own blood sugars while they are at school. These children may need to test their urine or blood for sugar levels before lunch, or they may need to eat at times other than the traditional lunch period. Adults who care for children with diabetes need to understand the disease. You need to know the signs and treatment for low blood sugar and when to call the doctor for help. Be sure to treat the child normally.

For more information about diabetes, contact the American Diabetes Association in your state or write the national organization.

American Diabetes Association National Service Center
1600 Duke St.
Alexandria, VA 22314
1-800-232-3472

Epilepsy

Epilepsy describes disorders of the central nervous system that are characterized by sudden and recurrent seizures. Seizures are abnormal discharges of electrical energy in the brain. Depending on the area of the brain involved, they can result in loss of consciousness, involuntary movements and/or abnormal motor movements or sensory experiences.

The three most common types of seizures that occur with epilepsy are grand mal, petit mal and psychomotor seizures.

A grand mal seizure, the most common type, involves both hemispheres of the brain. It causes violent shaking of the entire body, convulsions and loss of consciousness. The seizure usually lasts from two to five minutes. Grand mal seizures may occur several times a day or as infrequently as once a year.

Petit mal seizures are the most common type to occur in children. These seizures usually first occur between the ages of five and nine. They cause staring spells that last from five to twenty seconds. The seizures may occur infrequently or as often as a hundred times a day. Children with these seizures may look as if they are daydreaming or not paying attention.

Psychomotor seizures involve only one hemisphere of the brain. They cause inappropriate or purposeless behavior, including lengthy staring spells, aimless roaming or involuntary movements of parts of the body. The child does not lose consciousness, but during the seizure she or he will not be able to respond to the environment. The seizure usually lasts from two to five minutes. Psychomotor seizures may occur one or more times a week or once or twice a year.

The most common signs and symptoms of epilepsy include staring spells, tic-like movements, rhythmic movements of the head, purposeless sounds and body movements, head dropping, lack of response, eyes rolling upward, and chewing and swallowing movements. Watch for repeated occurrences of two or more of these symptoms happening together and without variation.

For more information about epilepsy, contact the Epilepsy Foundation of America in your state or write the national organization.

I Don't Feel Good

Epilepsy Foundation of America
4351 Garden City Dr., Suite 406
Landover, MD 20785
1-800-332-1000

Heart Conditions

A variety of heart conditions can affect children. Conditions that occur at birth from a defect in the formation of the heart are called *congenital heart defects*. Other conditions such as rheumatic heart disease may develop as a complication of an illness.

By the time children are four years old, most congenital heart defects will have been detected and corrected. A child with an undetected heart defect may look bluish (indicating lack of oxygen in the blood), especially around the lips and nailbeds. The child may squat during exercise to catch his or her breath. Children who have uncorrected congenital heart defects may need modified programs while they are in daycare or school.

Rheumatic heart disease is a preventable heart condition. However, children who do not receive needed antibiotics when they have strep throat may be susceptible to rheumatic fever, which can lead to rheumatic heart disease. A child with a questionable sore throat should be examined by a physician to determine if the sore throat is caused by the streptococcus bacteria, the culprit in rheumatic fever. Complications from rheumatic fever can result in damage to the heart valves.

For more information about the many types of heart defects and diseases seen in children, contact the American Heart Association in your state or write the national office.

American Heart Association National Center
7320 Greenville Ave.
Dallas, TX 75231-4599
1-800-242-1793

HIV/AIDS

AIDS, acquired immune deficiency syndrome, is a serious disease that is **not common** in children under ten years old. However, because of the seriousness of the disease and the fear it creates, a discussion of AIDS is important in a book on health conditions of children.

AIDS is a disease caused by the **Human Immunodeficiency Virus (HIV)**. The virus weakens the immune system, leaving the infected person vulnerable to many unusual and life-threatening illnesses. As the immune system weakens over time, the body becomes less able to fight off infection. Something as minor as a common cold can be very serious for a person who does not have an immune system to fight the infection.

At present, there is no cure for the disease. Drugs that are being developed are designed to help the immune system fight the infections that cause the person to be so ill. Most people who die with AIDS die from an "opportunistic infection" and not from the virus itself. The most commonly identified opportunistic infections are *Pneumocystis carinii* pneumonia (PCP), Kaposi's sarcoma, AIDS dementia, and wasting away syndrome.

The total number of AIDS cases in children under the age of twelve is about 2 percent of the total number of AIDS cases in the United States. At the end of 1990, the Centers for Disease Control reported approximately 2,600 cases of pediatric AIDS. However, this number only indicates those children who have symptoms that meet the definition of AIDS. Many children infected with the virus that causes AIDS, the Human Immunodeficiency Virus (HIV), do not show symptoms and are not ill.

Children under ten who are infected with HIV are vulnerable to infection when attending daycare or school. In most cases, the actual threat is to the child with the HIV infection from other children and their illnesses and not from the child with the disease. If an infected child is attending daycare or school, he or she may need to stay home during epidemics of chickenpox or flu to avoid being exposed to these diseases that may weaken the immune system.

I Don't Feel Good

HIV/AIDS

Determining whether a child with an HIV infection can attend daycare or school is usually decided on a case-by-case basis. Some state and local education agencies have committees that make recommendations regarding school attendance. However, the National Association of State Boards of Education (NASBE) suggests that having a committee make the decision may be disruptive to the school community and cause needless trauma for infected persons and their families. As an alternative, they recommend that "the superintendent follow a standard procedure to ensure the safety of persons in the school setting and to plan to support the person with the illness.... Unless there is a secondary infection that constitutes a medically recognized risk of transmission in the school setting, the superintendent shall not alter the education program of the infected person" (Fraser, 1989, p.10). NASBE further recommends that if the child is excluded, the plan for education "shall have minimal impact on education....It must be medically, legally, educationally, and ethically sound" (ibid.).

HIV infection is not easy to get. Today, most children under ten who are infected with Human Immunodeficiency Virus (HIV) will have been infected before or during birth from an infected mother. Mothers may have been infected in any of the ways that HIV can be contracted. (The most common means of getting the virus are through the exchange of blood or semen when sharing needles in IV drug use or having sex with an infected person.)

There may be some children in school who contracted the disease through blood transfusions. However, since 1985, all blood is tested to prevent the spread of the disease though receiving blood. The virus cannot be spread by sharing toys, hugging, or from a kiss, clothes or toilets.

The virus is very fragile and cannot live outside the human body for very long. As Quackenbush and Villarreal describe in their book *"Does AIDS Hurt?"* (Network Publications, 1988) a person must have very intimate and direct contact with the semen, vaginal secretions, blood or feces of an infected person for the virus to be transmitted. In the school setting, transmission of the virus would not be very likely except for the possibility of contact with blood from injuries on the playground. Children should be

HIV/AIDS

taught not to touch someone else's blood, but to call a grownup to help if someone is hurt.

If a daycare worker or teacher needs to clean up blood, urine or other body fluids, he or she should wear vinyl or latex gloves and clean the area with a 1:10 solution of bleach. As added prevention of the disease as well as all communicable diseases, the hands should be washed with soap and water.

For more information about AIDS, call your local AIDS hotline, the National AIDS Hotline or write the National AIDS Network (NAN).

National AIDS hotline: 1-800-342-AIDS (7 days a week, 24 hours a day)

National AIDS Network (NAN)
1012 14th St. NW
Suite 601
Washington, DC 20005
Telephone: 202-347-0390

Although chronic diseases are not common in children, at some time most caregivers and teachers will work with children who have one of these conditions or diseases. Knowing something about the disease and where to get more information can help you plan appropriate care and programs.

Many free or inexpensive materials are available from the organizations listed in this chapter. These materials can help teachers, caregivers and parents understand and handle children's chronic conditions. Other resources are available from local agencies; check your local phone book. Many state voluntary and public agencies have toll-free numbers for information. Contact the toll-free number information operator in your area by dialing 1-800-555-1212.

Note: Information in this chapter was taken from handouts and publications available from the voluntary agencies referred to in this chapter. Contact the agency for a list of current publications.

I Don't Feel Good

Appendix A

Sample Letters to Parents

The following are samples of letters that might be sent to parents by daycare and school officials concerning specific diseases that occur in the school setting. The letters may be used to educate parents about the disease, and tell what to do if their child contracts it. The information is taken from the text and can be easily adapted to meet personal needs.

Chickenpox

Dear Parents,

Chickenpox has been reported at your child's school. Chickenpox is a highly contagious viral disease that is very common in children. Please note the following signs and symptoms of the disease, and follow the recommended suggestions for preventing the spread of the disease to others.

Signs and Symptoms

- The day before the chickenpox rash appears, the child may be tired, run a slight fever and complain of a headache.

- The rash usually first appears on the back and neck and then spreads to the face and limbs. The flat red rash becomes raised, looking somewhat like insect bites, and then develops into small blisters.

- When the tiny blisters, called vesicles, break, the sores crust over. The sores are usually very itchy and are easily broken when scratched. New sores appear in stages for two to six days.

- While the child is breaking out with the vesicles, she or he may run a fever. After all the crusts have formed, the fever usually goes away.

Suggestions for Parents

- If your child has the signs and symptoms of chickenpox, keep him or her away from other people until all the blisters have crusted over.

- To help reduce the fever and to make the child more comfortable, many physicians recommend acetaminophen. **Do not give aspirin to a child with chickenpox** because of the possibility of contracting Reye's syndrome.

- Warm baths with baking soda (1/2 cup for each tub of water) may help reduce the itching. Calamine lotion can also be used to relieve the itching. If the itching is severe, the doctor may prescribe an antihistamine.

Cutting the child's fingernails and having the child wear gloves can reduce the chances of scarring from scratching.

- Keep the hands and skin clean. Handwashing is very important to prevent the spread of the infection or bacterial infections that may occur from scratching.

- The child may return to school a minimum of seven days after the rash has appeared and when all the blisters have crusted over.

Thank you for your cooperation.

_____

(Name of Principal, School Nurse or Teacher)

Head Lice

Dear Parents,

Head lice have been reported at your child's school. Please check your child for any of the following signs and symptoms. If your child is infected, follow the recommended suggestions for treatment and guidelines for returning to school.

Signs and Symptoms

Lice are small bloodsucking insects that attach to the hair and feed off the blood vessels in the scalp. You may see the lice in the hair near the scalp if you look carefully, or you might be able to see them with a magnifying glass.

Small nits or egg cases will be attached to the hair. The nits look like dandruff, except dandruff can be easily removed from the hair shaft while lice nits cannot.

The child's head may itch. There may also be small red bites resembling a rash on the scalp and behind the ears and neck.

Suggestions for Parents

- If your child has head lice, remain calm and treat the condition.

- Purchase an over-the-counter medication for lice. Lice medications come in the form of shampoo or creme rinse. Follow the directions as recommended on the label. Some of the medications you can purchase at the pharmacy or drugstore are NIX, A200 and RID.

- Comb out all the nits with the fine-tooth comb that is provided in most lice treatment packages. If one is not provided, you will need to purchase a fine-tooth comb to comb out the nits. The major reason lice come back is because all the nits are not combed out.

- At the same time you treat the hair, wash all bed linens, towels, brushes and head apparel in hot, soapy water.

- Place all objects that cannot be washed, such as stuffed animals, in plastic bags for ten days.

- Check other members of your household for head lice and treat them if necessary.

- Recheck your child's head for the presence of lice or nits for the next ten days. Some treatments may need to be repeated a second time.

- In severe cases of lice, consult your physician. There are stronger prescription medications that you may need to use.

- You may send your child back to school after the hair has been treated and when all the nits are gone.

Thank you for your cooperation.

_____

(Name of Principal, School Nurse or Teacher)

Influenza

Dear Parents,

Several children in your child's school have been sick with influenza. Flu is an infectious disease of the respiratory tract that lasts up to seven days and occasionally longer. Please check your child for any of the following signs and symptoms. If your child is infected, follow the recommended suggestions for treatment and guidelines for returning to school.

Signs and Symptoms

Influenza usually starts with a sudden onset of fever, followed by a severe cough, chills, headache and general achiness.

Suggestions for Parents

- For fever, headache and the general achiness associated with influenza, doctors may recommend acetaminophen. **Do not give aspirin to a child with influenza,** because it may lead to complications, including Reye's syndrome.

- A cool-mist humidifier may help relieve coughing.

- Gargling with salt water can help relieve the pain of sore throat. Mix one teaspoon of salt in one cup of warm water for gargling.

- Encourage the child to drink plenty of fluids.

- If the child develops rapid breathing, ear pain, a severe sore throat or symptoms that last more than seven days, call your doctor.

- Physical exertion should be discouraged while the symptoms persist.

- Your child should not return to school until all the symptoms are gone.

Thank you for your cooperation.

_____

(Name of Principal, School Nurse or Teacher)

Appendix B

Over-the-Counter Drugs for Common Skin Conditions

Skin Problem	Medication
Mosquito Bites*	hydrocortisone cream, calamine lotion
Fleas*	hydrocortisone cream, calamine lotion
Chiggers*	hydrocortisone cream, calamine lotion, Chiggerex
Spiders*	See Chapter 2
Ticks*	See Chapter 2
Bees/Wasp-like Insects*	Benadryl, sting kits
Lice*	NIX, A200, RID
Impetigo	triple antibiotic ointment
Ringworm	Tinactin, Lotrimin
Canker Sores	Gly-Oxide, Anbesol, Orabase
Fever Blisters	Blistex, Carmex, Campho Phenique, Anbesol

* For specific information on insect bites, refer to Chapter 2. Certain bites may require attention from a physician.

Appendix C

Procedure for Keeping an Airway Open

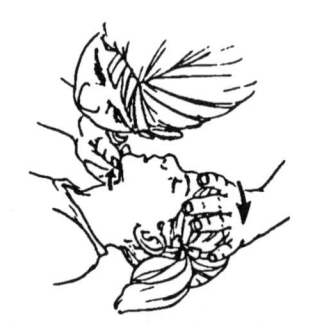

Kneel beside child's shoulder; lift the chin up gently with one hand while pushing down on the forehead with the other to tilt the head back into a sniffing or neutral position. The chin should be lifted so that the teeth are brought almost together. Avoid completely closing the mouth.

Reproduced with Permission. Textbook of Pediatric Basic Life Support. American Heart Association, 1988.

Appendix D

Recommended Schedule for Active Immunization of Normal Infants and Children

Age	Immunization
2 months	Haemophilus DTP (Diptheria, Tetanus and Pertussis) OPV (Oral Polio Virus)
4 months	Haemophilus DTP OPV
6 months	Haemophilus DTP OPV (may be given in geographical areas with increased risk of polio exposure)
15 months	Haemophilus MMR (Measles, Mumps, Rubella); tuberculin testing may also be done
18 months	DTP OPV
4–6 years	DTP OPV (at or before school entry)
11–12 years	MMR
14–16 years	Adult tetanus toxoid (full dose) and diptheria toxoid (reduced dose) in combination; repeat every 10 years throughout life

Adapted with permission from Immunization Protects Children.©1991. American Academy of Pediatrics.

References

American Academy of Pediatrics. 1987. *School health: A guide for health professionals.* Elk Grove Village, IL.

American Public Health Association. 1990. *Control of communicable diseases in man.* Washington, DC.

Fraser, K. 1989. *Someone at school has AIDS.* Alexandria, VA: National Association of State Boards of Education.

Lewis, K. D. and H. B. Thomson. 1986. *Manual of school health.* Reading, MA: Addison-Wesley.

Newton, J. 1984. *School health handbook. A ready reference for school nurses and educators.* Englewood Cliffs, NJ: Prentice-Hall.

Suggested Readings

American Red Cross. 1988. *American Red Cross Standard First Aid Workbook.*

Brazelton, B. T. 1989. *Toddlers and Parents.* New York: Doubleday.

Brazelton, B. T. 1990. *Families: Crisis and Caring.* New York: Ballantine Books.

Curwin, R. L. and A. N. Mendler. 1990. *Am I in Trouble? Using Discipline to Teach Young Children Responsibility.* Santa Cruz, CA: ETR Associates.

Mendler, A. N. 1990. *Smiling at Yourself: Educating Young Children About Stress and Self-Esteem.* Santa Cruz, CA: ETR Associates.

Pantell, R. H., J. F. Fries and D. M. Vickery. 1990. *Taking Care of Your Child: A Parent's Guide to Medical Care.* 3d ed. Reading, MA: Addison-Wesley.

An excellent manual for parents that provides advice on hundreds of common medical problems from birth to adolescence. The book includes more than 100 decision charts to help parents make decisions about the care of their children. Home remedies and descriptions of what to expect at the doctor's office are also provided.

Parcel, G. S. and C. E. Rinear. 1990. *Basic Emergency Care of the Sick and Injured.* 4th ed. St. Louis: Times-Mirror/Mosby.

Quackenbush, M. and S. Villarreal. 1988. *Does AIDS Hurt? Educating Young Children About AIDS.* Santa Cruz, CA: ETR Associates.

Scheer, J. K. 1990. *Germ Smart: Children's Activities in Disease Prevention.* Santa Cruz, CA: ETR Associates.

Thygerson, A. L. 1986. *The First Aid Book.* 2d ed. Englewood Cliffs, NJ: Prentice-Hall.

Your Child's Health Record, available from MetLife, is a free pamphlet that can help you keep track of all-important statistics about your child. The four-page booklet provides space to record information from your child's routine health checkups, including height, weight, blood pressure and doctor's comments; blood type; immunization and test dates; and family history of diseases. Also included is the immunization schedule recommended by the American Academy of Pediatrics. For a copy, send a self-addressed, stamped, business-sized envelope to Metropolitan Life, Health and Safety Education (16UV), Box HR, One Madison Ave., New York, NY 10010.

Child Health Record from Infancy to Adulthood, available from the American Academy of Pediatrics, is a booklet that helps parents keep track of health statistics of their children. It includes recommendations for health supervision of your child and spaces to record information such as pediatricians' names and addresses, family and newborn history, physical examination reports, developmental landmarks, immunizations, illnesses, dental reports, health notes and height and weight with charts. The booklet is available from the American Academy of Pediatrics, 141 Northwest Point Blvd., P.O. Box 927, Elk Grove Village, IL 60009-0927.

About the Author

Jane W. Lammers, EdD, CHES, is a professor of health education at the University of Central Arkansas in Conway, Arkansas. She has worked with teachers, school nurses and administrators for the past ten years, dealing with the issues of health appraisal of the school-age child in a yearly college course. She serves on the Arkansas Advisory Council for the Southwest Regional Center for Drug-Free Schools and Communities and is a member of the Summit Team, a policy-making advisory group for drug prevention. Since 1983, with a grant from the Arkansas Division of Alcohol and Drug Abuse Prevention, she has conducted yearly evaluation on the effects of a comprehensive school health education curriculum on the prevention of drug abuse among elementary school children. She has published numerous articles in health education journals and has made presentations in all areas of health education.

Tackle Today's Tough Issues With More Practical Handbooks

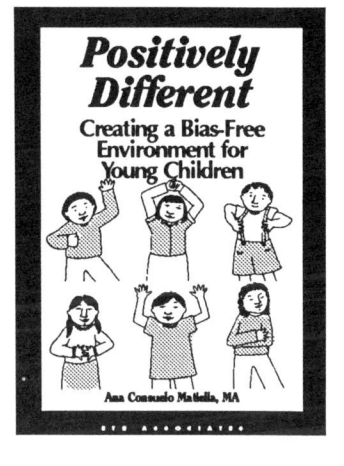

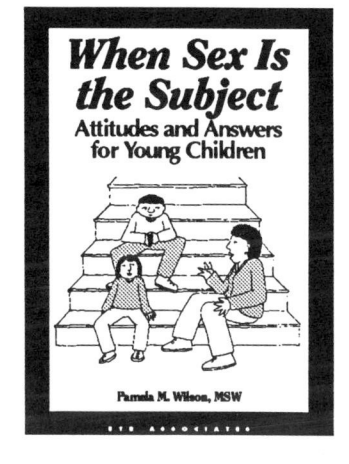

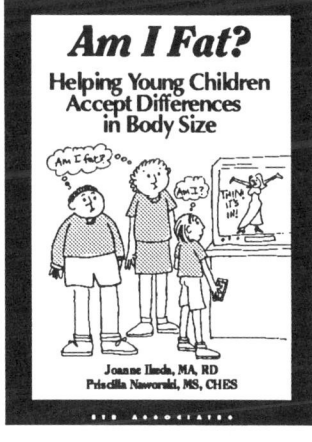

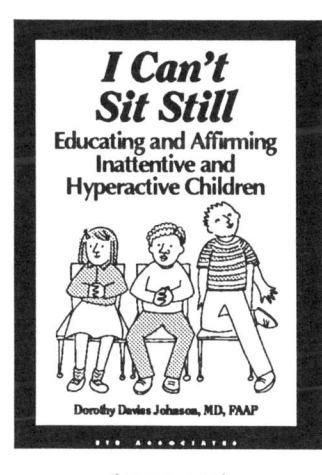

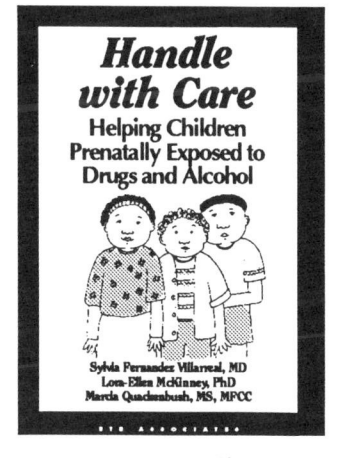

Positively Different
Creating a Bias-Free Environment for Young Children
Ana Consuelo Matiella, MA
(#509-H1)

When Sex Is the Subject
Attitudes and Answers for Young Children
Pamela M. Wilson, MSW
(#583-H1)

Am I Fat?
Helping Young Children Accept Differences in Body Size
Joanne Ikeda, MA, RD
Priscilla Naworski, MS, CHES
(#569-H1)

I Can't Sit Still
Educating and Affirming Inattentive and Hyperactive Children
Dorothy Davies Johnson, MD, FAAP
(#560-H1)

Handle with Care
Helping Children Prenatally Exposed to Drugs and Alcohol
Sylvia Fernandez Villarreal, MD
Lora-Ellen McKinney, PhD
Marcia Quackenbush, MS, MFCC
(#594-H1)

Learn a variety of positive, hands-on approaches to help children up to age ten understand the health issues that shape their lives. The Issues Books from ETR Associates. For more information and a complete list of Issues Books...

Call Toll-Free 1 (800) 321-4407

or contact:
**Sales Department
ETR Associates**
P.O. Box 1830
Santa Cruz, CA 95061-1830
FAX: (408) 438-4284